C0-AWB-479

Containing Costs in Third Party Drug Programs

Selected Bibliography and Abstracts

David A. Knapp, Ph.D.

and Francis B. Palumbo, Ph.D.

One in a series of studies and reports made possible by a grant from Roche Laboratories, a division of Hoffmann-La Roche Inc.

Containing Costs in Third Party Drug Programs

Selected Bibliography and Abstracts

David A. Knapp, Ph.D.
Professor and Chairman
Department of Pharmacy Administration
School of Pharmacy
University of Maryland at Baltimore

and Francis B. Palumbo, Ph.D.
Assistant Professor of Pharmacy Administration
School of Pharmacy
University of Maryland at Baltimore

DRUG INTELLIGENCE PUBLICATIONS, INC., HAMILTON, ILLINOIS 62341

LIBRARY OF CONGRESS CATALOG NUMBER 78-50224
ISBN 0-914768-28-x

Printed in the United States of America by

THE HAMILTON PRESS, INC., HAMILTON, ILLINOIS 62341

Foreword

Perhaps more quickly than any other segment of the provision of health care, pharmacy is moving to prepare for its role under national health insurance in the United States.

Certainly the costs of prescription drugs under such a program would be far less than those for hospital care or physician services. In the case of drugs, extreme differences between the views of providers and those of patients are apparently less serious. However, drug coverage under virtually any national insurance program would be marked by unique problems, complexities and disputes that call for the most careful consideration and analysis.

The study of drug insurance was given its major impetus by the appearance of the final report and the background papers of the HEW Task Force on Prescription Drugs in 1968 and 1969. When those reports were published, one of our distinguished colleagues told us, "Never again will the drug industry, or pharmacy, or the medical profession be the same."

Clearly, that prophecy has been fulfilled. During the past decade, remarkable alterations in the views toward drug use and drug insurance have been expressed by many leaders in industry, pharmacy and medicine. New policies have been proposed—and some have already been implemented.

At the same time, there has been an enormous proliferation of publications on all of the various aspects of drug use and drug insurance. Some of these publications are readily available, others are not. Some have appeared in pharmacy or medical journals, some in government papers, some in special monographs.

As a preliminary guide to such material, David Knapp and Francis Palumbo have prepared this annotated bibliography covering some 250 books and articles. It is, in part, a description of the state of the art. It is also a description of the state of the literature, mostly from 1970 to 1977.

The authors have elected to focus their attention on cost containment in any national drug insurance approach, and to present summaries rather than critiques of each publication. Few, if any, individuals in this country are more qualified to undertake such an analysis. Their bibliography will be invaluable to those in government who must make decisions and to those who will seek to influence the decisions.

Of particular importance, we believe, is the inclusion of material on the drug insurance programs in Canada, the United Kingdom, Australia, New Zealand and several countries in Western Europe. The lessons that can be learned from their experiences may not all be applicable to the United States, but it seems prudent that we be aware of them. If we are to make mistakes, let us not repeat those of other countries. At the very least, let our mistakes be original. And, if the goals of Drs. Knapp and Palumbo are achieved, such mistakes will be minimal.

San Francisco PHILIP R. LEE, M.D.

December 1977 MILTON SILVERMAN, Ph.D.

Preface

No topic in the health care field has received more attention in recent years than the skyrocketing costs of all components of medical care, including drugs. In their Foreword to this book, which we gratefully acknowledge, Silverman and Lee point to the importance of cost containment in any national drug insurance program. While undeniably true, cost containment issues are of interest not only to planners but also are immediately relevant to the administrators, clients and providers of the large number of third party drug programs already in existence.

This bibliography tries to bring together the relevant literature on cost containment in both public and private third party drug programs. Any selected bibliography such as this reflects the judgments of its authors and thus is subject to their biases and whims. The authors, therefore, are solely responsible for shortcomings in the list. Many, however, contributed to the development of the bibliography.

Roche Laboratories provided financial support for the project and Kwang Lee of Roche was an invaluable source of information and advice. We had the advantage of starting with an enormous and exhaustive bibliography prepared for Roche by Dr. Donald Yett of the University of Southern California. Winifred Sewell of the University of Maryland led us through the intricacies of bibliographic and abstracting mechanics, and abstractors Alice Bevan, Joy Kahn, Helen Mashbaum, and Sydney Schultz demonstrated an uncanny ability to distill the essence of the most complicated article or the longest book. Gwen Simmons, Phyllis Sivels and Lena Mitchell provided secretarial assistance, including the onerous task of accurately typing a 258-item bibliography!

At Drug Intelligence Publications, Inc., we benefited from

the advice and assistance of Dr. Donald E. Francke and his associates, including Harvey A. K. Whitney, Jr., Mary Ann Jaske, and Linda J. Dodds. To all of them, our thanks.

Baltimore DAVID A. KNAPP, Ph.D.

December 1977 FRANCIS B. PALUMBO, Ph.D.

Contents

Introduction and Organization

Third-party coverage of out-of-hospital prescribed drugs accounts for an increasing proportion of total drug expenditures in the United States. As programs covering drugs become larger, methods of cost containment become increasingly important, not only because of their impact on the programs themselves, but also because of their effect on the total market for prescribed drugs. As the debate over national health insurance progresses in the months and years to come, the shape of a potential drug benefit will depend to a great extent on how carefully cost containment mechanisms can be shaped.

There is a large literature bearing on the issue of cost containment in drug programs, but it is scattered in pharmacy and medical journals, health services research publications, public health periodicals, government documents and books. Despite the difficulty of obtaining information, it is important that workers in this field, particularly policy makers, be familiar not only with the "accepted truths" of the area, but also with the original literature. In this way, perhaps more informed judgments may be made.

It is the purpose of this publication to bring together a representative annotated bibliography of the literature related to cost containment in drug programs. All types of literature are included: books, pamphlets, journal articles, government documents and a few conference presentations. Excluded are most unsigned news articles and unpublished papers.

The bibliography primarily covers 1970 through August 1977. Some particularly useful earlier references, such as the reports of the Task Force on Prescription Drugs, have also been included. A wide variety of journals in medicine, pharmacy, public health, economics and business were searched, and an extensive bibliography provided by Roche Laboratories led to many additional sources.

This book consists of four main parts: the abstracts; the bibliography, or index of primary authors; an index of secondary authors; and a subject index.

The main portion of the book is devoted to the abstracts themselves, which are arranged by subject in the twelve chapters listed in the Table of Contents. The first four chapters make up

Section I, which deals with an overview of cost containment issues in both a drug and nondrug context. Items related to experiences in other countries and to inpatient settings are included here.

Section II, with eight chapters, is devoted to a subject-by-subject consideration of specific drug cost control approaches, including controls on patients, product cost, dispensing cost and prescriber behavior.

Within each chapter, abstracts are arranged first by year published, in reverse chronological order; and, within year, alphabetically by author. An abstract may appear in more than one chapter if it deals with more than one major topic.

Each abstract is headed by the title, followed by the abstract number. On right hand pages the abstract number is to the right; on left hand pages the abstract number is to the left. The text of the abstract follows next. Items were abstracted by specialists in library science and reviewed for content accuracy by the authors. The abstracts describe the contents of the original article or book, but are not intended to be critical reviews.

At the end of the abstract is the number of references cited in the original article. If part of the content of the abstract is relevant to the topic of other chapter(s), key words will appear next. The remainder of the citation then appears.

At the end of chapters 3–12, a list of cross-references is included, indexed to abstract number and page. Thus, if a reader wished to be complete in a search on a particular topic, the cross-references should also be examined.

The bibliography contains a complete literature citation of each item abstracted, arranged alphabetically by primary author. To the left of each citation is an unique abstract number; to the right of each citation is the number of the page on which the abstract appears. The unique abstract number is used throughout the book for cross-referencing purposes, but has no inherent meaning.

Next is an index of secondary authors keyed to primary authors and abstract numbers. Since the bibliography and the secondary author index are mutually exclusive, it would be necessary to search both lists to determine, for example, all publications authored by a specific person.

Finally, a subject index is provided. Although the abstracts themselves are arranged basically by subject, this index will aid in locating references to terms other than chapter titles or key words.

Section One

Cost Containment: An Overview

Included in this section are items which either deal with cost containment in a general way or which discuss a number of approaches to controlling drug costs. Also included are references to approaches in other countries or in inpatient settings.

I

General Aspects of Cost Containment

Items abstracted do not deal specifically with drugs or pharmacy services. No key word.

1976

Medicare-Medicaid: An Appraisal After Ten Years

13

A major portion of this issue of *Public Health Reports* is devoted to several papers on Medicare and Medicaid. Each article is briefly abstracted below.

Arthur E. Hess, in discussing a ten-year perspective on Medicare, notes coverage, accomplishments, cost and quality controls (including Professional Standards Review Organization legislation). He suggests that the Medicare experience can be applied to planning national health insurance. Coverage and eligibility requirements of Medicare/Medicaid should be adjusted to make Medicare the basic, comprehensive program providing a full range of hospital and medical services to the aged and, where possible, to the disabled. This leaves other services to Medicaid, such as long-term care and services to the nondisabled and nonaged poor.

In reflecting on a decade of Medicaid, M. Keith Weikel and Nancy A. LeaMond observe that Medicaid has improved the financial access of the poor to medical services and provides experience valuable in considering a national health insurance program. They discuss antecedents, major features, management problems and costs, and accomplishments of Medicaid.

Karen Davis reviews achievements and problems of Medicaid and attributes its high costs to an increase in the number of recipients covered under Aid to Families with Dependent Children, the rise in medical care prices and the high costs of nursing home care. She discusses trends in health care utilization and health status of the poor, and the inequitable distribution of benefits due to differences in state welfare eligibility. Reforms are suggested.

Discussing Medicare, medical practice and the medical profession, Ernest W. Saward makes note of the pre-Medicare climate, the effects on medical practice of Medicare controls, regulations and costs, and the public stance of the medical profession on priorities in the allocation of health resources.

Avedis Donabedian remarks on the effects of Medicare and Medicaid on access to, and quality of, health care. He discusses the increase in use of physicians and hospital services by the poor and suggests a greater exposure to the hazards of unnecessary and inappropriate medical care, but concludes that, overall, the poor are receiving more and better care.

Gordon McLachlin, of the Nuffield Provincial Hospitals of London, presents a British view of the United States under Medicaid and Medicare.

Finally, Walter J. McNerney, in a treatment of health insurance in the Medicare years, discusses developments in group health insurance, relations between government and the private insurance industry, cost containment, economic and social determinants of the health care climate (for example, consumer movements), areawide planning, utilization review and quality assessment, reimbursement and alternative delivery systems such as Health Maintenance Organizations (HMOs).

References, 69

ANONYMOUS. Special section of seven papers. *Public Health Reports 91* (4):299–342, July–August 1976. Pages 299–302, 303–308, 309–316, 317–321, 322–331, 332–335, 336–342.

Benefits in Medical Care Programs

54

Discusses the services included as benefits in medical care programs under several forms of prepayment. Reports both theory and empirical work for use in formulating policy, and planning and administering health care programs. Establishes principles and problems of introducing prepaid benefits in a medical care system, and discusses social action in the health field and utilization patterns of health care services. Deals with program objectives in terms of patients, organizations, providers and the social system. Finds deductible and copayment features to be effective means of reducing medical care costs. Reviews research showing that third-party insurance for prescription drugs is associated with more frequent dispensing of prescriptions and a small increase in the average charge per prescription. Suggests the substitutability of drugs and physician visits; when the number of physician visits is limited, more drugs are prescribed for a longer period of time. Appendices present a formula for deriving actual price and net price paid by insured for health-related services, and a health plan grading system (1000-point scale) based on administration, extent of coverage, scope of benefits, quality control and out-of-pocket costs.

References, 280. *Key words:* Patient cost sharing.

DONABEDIAN, AVEDIS. Cambridge, Massachusetts. Harvard University Press, 1976.

Issues in National Health Insurance

55

Proposals for national health insurance are described and analyzed within the framework of two opposing views of the present medical care system: (1) that the system is sound and growing and that the purpose of health insurance is to protect us from the unpredictable costs of illness, or (2) that the system is inefficient and inequitable and that national health insurance must not only protect us from the costs of illness but also reform the health care system. It is recognized that the ultimate national health insurance scheme is likely to be based on a compromise viewpoint. The effects of a health insurance plan are to lower consumer costs for the insured services, thus improving the ability to pay for non-insured services, and to produce a source of revenue for the health services providers. These effects lead to an increase in demand for certain types of services, resulting in increased prices.

The next step in this model is the demand for increased insurance coverage; thus the process "feeds upon itself." Consequences of eight components of a national health insurance plan—including cost control, efficiency of production and allocation, adequacy of coverage and geographic distribution of services—are predicted; some are desirable and some undesirable. To balance costs and benefits, national health insurance should include the following, graduated to income: a substantial deductible provision, copayment and a limit on annual out-of-pocket expenditures. Reform of the health care system is desirable through organizational changes and professional review mechanisms.

References, 12. *Key words:* Patient cost sharing.

DONABEDIAN, AVEDIS. *American Journal of Public Health 66* (4):345–350, April 1976.

The Problem of Rising Health Care Costs

59

Factors affecting health care costs and inflationary trends are analyzed from an economic rather than a social viewpoint. Prices rose substantially in fiscal 1975 for medical and hospital services, physicians' services and drugs, outpacing increases in the economy as a whole. Consumer price index data for 1965–75 are presented. The impact of this inflation on industry, labor, government and the individual is discussed, along with health care issues such as third-party payments, public and private health insurance financing, government support, the role of the physician, the incentive structure, technological change, wage and price controls and quality of medical care. Explanations for high health care costs to consumers include great increases in wages and prices for equipment and supplies, changes in health care services which require greater labor and nonlabor expenses, increased energy costs, and malpractice insurance premium increases and the related increase in the use of laboratory tests.

Studies suggest that third-party payment leads to greater consumer demand than if consumers were to bear the full cost of health care services. Since 80 per cent of health insurance premiums are paid through group plans, most consumers are unaware of medical insurance costs. Third-party payments in fiscal 1975 accounted for 67.4 per cent of total personal health care expenditures; private health insurance payments for 26.5 per cent. Payments for drugs are small but rising. Public funds (Federal, state, local) account for 42.2 per cent of total health expenditures. Public support is also available in the form of tax subsidies and exemptions for nonprofit hospitals and insurance plans. Since the providers of health care services determine the nature of those services, traditional economic supply/demand forces are not allowed to operate. Also, financial incentives seem to encourage quantity rather than quality of service (e.g., the fee-for-service concept) and there is limited price competition.

References, 16.

EXECUTIVE OFFICE OF THE PRESIDENT. Council on Wage and Price Stability staff report. *Medical Marketing and Media 11* (11):42–47, 50, 52, 54–59, November 1976.

From Bismarck To Woodcock: The "Irrational" Pursuit of National Health Insurance

72

In response to the endorsement of comprehensive national health insurance for the United States by Leonard Woodcock of the United Auto Workers' Union, Professor Fuchs endeavors to explain the popularity of national health insurance throughout the world from the time of Bismarck in Germany in the 19th century, and the manner in which it has served diverse interests. Reasons for the development of national health insurance programs have included societal benefits, such as the prevention of communicable diseases, egalitarianism, the decline of the family and the church as agencies of care and support for the sick, and the need for a national symbol for increasing allegiance.

Interest in national health insurance in the United States has lagged because of traditional distrust of government, heterogeneity of population, and greater equality of opportunity for social and economic betterment (which makes "achievers" less likely to feel an obligation for those less well off). Other considerations related to national health insurance in the United States include tax advantages, perceived government control over health service providers, and alternative sources of funds for medical care in the form of government-supported hospitals, philanthropy, and even the acceptance of bad debts.

References, 22.

FUCHS, VICTOR, R. *The Journal of Law and Economics* 19 (2):347–359, August 1976.

Strategies for Financing National Health Insurance: Who Wins and Who Loses

158

National health insurance can be funded by prepayments (premiums, payroll taxes and income taxes) and by some form of cost sharing such as copayments. The greater the proportion of financing through taxes, the greater the share of health care costs borne by higher-income groups. The economic impact of various financing models is discussed, and a combination of funding sources to effectively distribute health insurance costs is proposed. Most current proposals suggest prepayments to account for about 85 per cent of costs, and cost-sharing mechanisms for 15 per cent. Funds for prepayments have been estimated at two-thirds from premiums or payroll taxes and the remaining third from income taxes. Premiums for individuals are suggested at 40 per cent of the amount for families.

Health insurance programs financed primarily through premiums rather than payroll taxes are less discriminatory against single individuals. Payroll taxes, although paid wholly or partly by employers, are actually passed on to employees. A program funded by income taxes places a relatively high financial burden on upper-income families. It is suggested that eliminating cost sharing for lower-income families would increase demand for services, thus adding to total costs and, consequently, to the financial burden of middle- and higher-income families.

Models for equitable distribution of these expenses, using combinations of payroll taxes or premiums with income taxes, plus uniform or reduced copayment and deductible provisions for lower-income families, are examined. Additional financial considerations involve tax exemptions for health insurance premiums, and deductions allowed for medical expenses.

References, 4. *Key words:* Patient cost sharing.

MITCHELL, BRIDGER M.; and SCHWARTZ, WILLIAM B. *New England Journal of Medicine* 295 (16):866–871, October 14, 1976.

Health: United States 1975

163

Presents statistics on national health expenditure trends since 1929, sources of funds for health expenditures (reflecting a shift from private to public sources), allocation of health expenditures, health manpower and health facilities, and health status and use of health services. Nearly 90 per cent of all hospital expenses involved third-party payments, but only 14 per cent of dental and drug expenses were covered in 1974.

References, not counted; footnotes used.

NATIONAL CENTER FOR HEALTH STATISTICS. Health Resources Administration. DHEW Publication No. (HRA) 76-1232. Washington, D.C., U.S. Government Printing Office, 1976.

Forward Plan for Health–FY 1978–1982

247

Major health care issues—costs, quality of care, research and development, health care delivery systems—are discussed, and recommendations made for a cohesive political, social and economic approach to health care problems. Goals include both meeting health care needs and improving the responsiveness of federal health-related research and administrative agencies. Cost containment proposals include strengthening state and local planning and development of health care resources, providing for better geographic and specialty distribution of health care personnel and equipment, reducing reimbursement problems and imbalances, encouraging the use of outpatient care where appropriate, supporting the Maximum Allowable Cost program to contain prescription drug costs, and implementing Professional Standards Review Organizations (PSROs) and other measures to reduce inappropriate use of health care services.

Specific topics examined include Health Maintenance Organizations, prospective rather than retrospective reimbursement, cost-sharing plans, improving consumer awareness of health care costs and reform of Medicaid/Medicare programs. Other proposals deal with preventive health care measures to improve the health of children, foster better nutritional practices and control environmental toxins. Health-related legislation and developments for fiscal year 1976 are reviewed, and data are presented on various aspects of the general health of the United States population. For example, the percentage of national health expenditures for drugs and drug sundries has declined from 16.7 per cent in 1929 to 8.9 per cent in 1975. Third-party payments for personal health care have increased from 11.5 per cent in 1929 to 67.4 per cent in 1975.

References, not counted; footnotes used. *Key words:* Maximum allowable cost.

U.S. DEPARTMENT OF HEALTH, EDUCATION, AND WELFARE, PUBLIC HEALTH SERVICE. Washington, D.C., The Department, August 1976.

1975

Will Shortages of Raw Materials and Rising Prices Hurt Our Chances for Better Health Care?

125

Current and projected world economic situations are described, and recommendations made for action by health professionals to maintain and improve health care by dealing with (1) conditions of economic stability and re-alignment of wealth and political power, (2) rising prices, and (3) shortages of energy, petrochemicals and other raw materials.

These problems affect health care in several ways: rising costs for oil, gas and electrical utilities, rising expectations leading to demands for better health care services, shortages of plastics products such as disposable syringes and intravenous tubing, shortages of organic solvents used for extracting drugs, shortages of paper products. Health service leaders and hospital administrators should institute conservation and recycling programs in existing and future facilities, upgrade maintenance practices, foster cooperative arrangements among area hospitals and encourage interdisciplinary dialogue. A National Health Planning Council for Energy and Materials is proposed.

References, 20.

KLINE, A. BURT. *Public Health Reports 90* (*1*):3–9, January–February 1975.

1963

An Evaluation of Administrative Controls in Medical Care Programs

56

Good medical care depends on (1) professionalization (settings which maximize the operation of professional criteria, incentives and goals), and (2) organization (so that professional personnel become responsive to administrative goals while preserving autonomy of patient care). Administrative control is required to maintain budgetary, legal and operational limits, but is difficult where providers of services are not full-time salaried personnel utilizing an agency's own facilities. In other words, control is difficult for health insurance and public-welfare medical care where there can be only partial control of physicians' services. Categories of control are (1) participation of recipients and providers of services, to assure quality of care and for reasons of economy and efficiency, (2) utilization of services, to cope with fluctuations in demand, (3) remuneration of providers of services and control of total costs, made difficult by the fee-for-service system, and (4) conduct or quality of professional activities.

Participation of recipients may be limited by personal factors such as age, residence, veteran status, disability or disease, economic status, group membership, or waiting periods. However, social objectives should not be compromised in determining administrative control. Participation of providers of service is determined by professional qualifications, such as licensure, professional society membership, or specialty board certification. Utilization is controlled by precise definition of benefits, exclusions and maximum payments. Deductibles and copayments may deter suspected areas of overutilization. A program may refuse to approve services to patients unless recommended by a physician. Also, some programs require that recipients certify that professional services were received. Review programs must not hinder provision of services.

Studies suggest greater hospitalization and surgery for fee-for-service insurance remuneration than for prepaid group practices, but the factor of professional judgment presents difficulties for administrative control. Administrative control of costs can be maintained by methods of payment for providers (annual salaries, fee schedules, or flat-rate payments, although it is difficult to determine professional fees rationally), continuous verification of expenditures, and limiting financial responsibility. Professional care can be controlled by minimum standards for acceptable care and by offering benefits that promote judicious utilization. Periodic administrative and professional review programs are required. The administering agency is responsible for defining goals, determining services and the manner in which they are rendered, and maintaining fiscal integrity and quality of care. A system combining administrative and professional control over the provision of health care services is recommended.

References, 41. *Key words:* Patient cost sharing, reimbursement.

DONABEDIAN, AVEDIS; and ATTWOOD, JULIA C. *New England Journal of Medicine* 269 (7):347–354, August 15 1963.

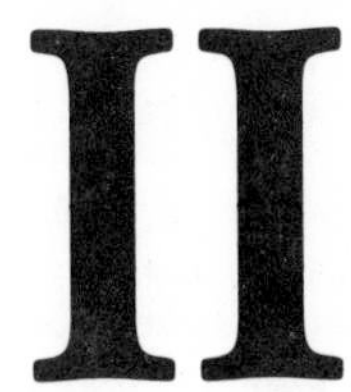

Controlling Costs in Drug Programs

Items included deal with the overall aspects of cost control in drug programs, or deal in depth with multiple approaches to cost containment. No key word.

1977

The Mysteries of Prescription Pricing in Retail Pharmacies

21

This study involved a two-week sample of retail drug prices from 20 pharmacies in a large midwestern city.

A review of more than 13,000 prescriptions for 100 representative drug products revealed substantial price variations among pharmacies and within the same pharmacy for the study period. These unpredictable pricing practices serve to discourage rational purchasing behavior on the part of consumers. For example, prices for 25 tetracycline hydrochloride 250 mg ranged from $1.37 to $4.51. Differences in mark-up could account for this inter-pharmacy price variation. The highest percentage mark-up among the 15 most frequently prescribed drugs was 92.8 per cent, for erythromycin 250 mg. Within the same pharmacy, prices for the identical prescription varied as much as 130 per cent. With one exception, it was not possible to classify the pharmacies as consistently low or high in drug prices. The data do not support the suggestion that the price variation can be explained by self-paying versus insured consumers.

References, 7.

BERKI, S.E.; RICHARDS, J.W.; and WEEKS, H.A. *Medical Care 15* (3):241–250, March 1977.

Annual Prescription Survey by the Albany College of Pharmacy

49

This paper analyzes the 1976 survey data concerning generic prescriptions, prescription costs and other cost data, frequency of particular drugs prescribed, frequency of drug therapeutic class prescribed, and frequency of dosage forms prescribed. This prescription audit consists of 15,031 prescriptions from 99 community pharmacies, located primarily in New York.

Some of the significant data discussed in detail are: (1) the 200 most frequently prescribed drugs, (2) the manufacturers of these 200 drugs, (3) the top 20 generic drugs, (4) a 10-year profile of generic prescriptions as a percentage of all new drugs, (5) the top 25 nonlegend drugs, (6) a 10-year comparison of prescription costs, and (7) a 10-year profile of the frequency distribution of drugs in various cost categories paid by the general public and by Medicaid.

Several of the significant finds are: (1) diazepam was the most frequently prescribed drug for the fifth consecutive year, (2) Roche Laboratories manufactured 11.5 per cent of the 200 most frequently prescribed drugs, (3) the average prescription price was $5.22, (4) generic prescriptions accounted for 13.1 per cent of the top 200 drugs and for 12.7 per cent of all new prescriptions, (5) ampicillin is the generic drug most frequently prescribed, and (6) antibiotics make up the therapeutic class most frequently prescribed (18.3%).

References, 0. *Key words:* Drug utilization review, substitution.

DENUZZO, RINALDO V. *Medical Marketing and Media 12* (4):32–43, 46, 48–49, April 1977.

Drug Cost Control: The Road to the Maximum Allowable Cost Regulations

73

Reviews the more than 15 years of Congressional investigation of the pharmaceutical industry and the increasing involvement of the federal government in financing health care programs, as background to the development of the Maximum Allowable Cost (MAC) regulations on drug costs.

The Kefauver hearings (1959–62), the Nelson hearings (1967–), the HEW Task Force on Prescription Drugs (1967–69), and the Kennedy hearings (1973–), all focused attention on the lack of price competition for pharmaceuticals fostered by the 17-year period of patent protection for new drugs. However, growing interest in generic prescribing is encouraging price competition for multisource drugs. This has led to a controversy over chemical and therapeutic equivalence of drug products and standards for drug quality, and criticism of the consistently high profits in the pharmaceutical industry, notwithstanding legitimate research and development expenditures. 1962 legislation required proof of efficacy for new drug products and 1972 legislation limited physician and hospital charges and established Professional Standards Review Organizations for Medicare/Medicaid programs.

Two approaches to drug cost control have been considered: (1) utilization review, and (2) more cost-effective reimbursement programs. Utilization review studies reveal problems such as inappropriate prescribing and adverse drug reactions. Cost effectiveness studies focus on copayment programs. Thus, the need to improve cost effectiveness in Medicare/Medicaid programs led to the development of the MAC regulations, including mechanisms for reviewing bioequivalence through the FDA and for setting price limits on multisource drugs through the Pharmaceutical Reimbursement Board and the Pharmaceutical Reimbursement Advisory Committee. In addition, HEW will provide information on costs of frequently prescribed drugs in order to assist states in estimating actual cost to the pharmacist of prescription drugs rather than retail cost, for use as the basis for reimbursement. The success of such procedures for drug cost containment is seen as having considerable impact on the future of national health insurance legislation.

References, 34. *Key words:* Drug utilization review, patient cost sharing.

FULDA, THOMAS R. *In* Friedman, Kenneth; and Rakoff, Stuart. *Toward a National Health Policy. Public Policy in the Control of Health Care Costs.* Lexington, Massachusetts, Lexington Books, 1977. Pages 55–67.

Categorically Needy and Medically Needy. Drug Utilization Among the Aged and Disabled

123

Drug utilization patterns by Medicaid patients were discussed for fourteen therapeutic classes. The program reviewed had no copayment feature and no formulary, and the utilization patterns observed could be attributed to differences in the patient subgroups studied. These Medicaid subgroups were: (1) categorically needy (CN), old age assistance (AA) and aid to the disabled (AD), and (2) medically needy (MN), both AA and AD. Over 1,200,000 prescriptions were examined.

The major findings were: (1) in each of the fourteen categories, except tranquilizers, the MN-AA group used more drugs than the CN-AA patients, and (2) the MN-AD patients used more drugs in all categories than the CN-AD group. Persons within the MN group tended to have more severe or chronic diseases than those in the CN group. Data were also analyzed for each group by expenditures for each therapeutic class when compared to expenditures for a base group, hypotensive agents. Finally, the differences in expenditure patterns between AA and AD categories were presented. These aid categories tended to be a more uniform determinant of utilization patterns than aid groups MN and CN, when measured by expenditures by therapeutic class and by expenditures per eligible patient. The usefulness of the data to Medicaid administrators was discussed.

References, 18. *Key words:* Drug utilization review.

KENNARD, LON; LAVENTURIER, MARC; and LANG, CHERYL. *Medical Marketing and Media 12* (2):31, 34, 36–38, February 1977.

The Task Force on Prescription Drugs: A Review of Problems, Progress and Possibilities

145

The chairman of the Task Force on Prescription Drugs, which was in existence from 1967 to 1969, assesses the impact of the recommendations of the Task Force after seven years. The major recommendation of the report was to include an outpatient drug benefit under Medicare. Although legislation to accomplish this has been introduced into the Congress on several occasions, it has yet to be accomplished. The most serious question related to this sort of coverage is the efficient administration of a drug benefit. Discussion now seems to be shifting to a consideration of an outpatient drug benefit under a national health insurance scheme. This would involve coverage for the 2.8

billion prescriptions dispensed in 1975 at a total cost of 14 billion dollars. In addition, another 4.5 billion dollars was spent for non-prescription medications.

A second major recommendation of the Task Force was to permit the federal government to set up reasonable cost ranges for drug products paid for under government programs. Progress in this area has been made through the Maximum Allowable Cost program. A third recommendation suggested the publication of a federal drug compendium which would supplant and replace package inserts and the *Physicians' Desk Reference.* This recommendation has been carried out.

Other less controversial recommendations have resulted in action in the last few years. For example, a national drug code has been established and the concept of drug use review is now widely recognized and institutionalized through the Professional Standards Review Organization legislation. Finally, the bioequivalency controversy has become somewhat less emotional over the last few years. In summary, it appears that the Task Force was able to have a significant effect on public policy in the drug field because of support of its recommendations from both Democratic and Republican administrations.

References, 5. *Key words:* Drug utilization review, maximum allowable cost. See abstract 244, page 50.

LEE, PHILIP R. *Drug Information Journal 11* (*1*):7–10, March 1977.

Drug Coverage under National Health Insurance: The Policy Options

217 Developing a plan for drug coverage under national health insurance is one of the most complicated matters facing health policy makers today. This monograph seeks to describe drug coverage in current programs, including commercial insurance plans, federal programs, state Medicaid programs, and national programs in six foreign countries. In addition, a tabulation of the specifics of drug coverage in pending federal legislation is included. Detailed background information is provided on a variety of drug-related topics such as rational prescribing, the use of generics, formularies, drug utilization review, data processing and cost controls.

An extensive portion of the monograph is devoted to a critical analysis of nine major policy areas in which decisions need to be made in any national health insurance program. These include:

1. selection of beneficiaries,
2. selection of covered drug products (formularies, product selection),
3. cost sharing by patients,
4. reimbursement of product cost,
5. reimbursement of dispensing cost,
6. alternative reimbursement approaches,
7. reimbursement methods,
8. data processing, and
9. utilization review.

A 98-item bibliography is included.

References, not counted; footnotes used.

SILVERMAN, MILTON; and LYDECKER, MIA. NCHSR. Research Report Series. DHEW Publication No. (HRA) 77-3189. Springfield, Virginia, National Technical Information Service, 1977.

Results of Medicaid Provider Review—Massachusetts

231

The Medicaid Examiner Program, developed by DHEW to combat state fraud and abuse, conducted its first review jointly with the Commonwealth of Massachusetts Department of Public Welfare, beginning June 15, 1976. The quality of medical services rendered was not at issue; the review's purpose was to detect claims discrepancies and to suggest changes in program structure and reimbursement methods to combat such abuses. Reviewed were 53 physicians, 50 pharmacies and 9 clinical laboratories; half of the physicians were selected because records showed a greater than average number of lab tests and services per patient and a greater than average amount paid per patient by the Massachusetts Medicaid program.

Computer profiles of recipients' medical histories and service providers' billing records were examined; 25 paid claims for each provider were selected for review. Physician abuses found included discrepancies between services billed and rendered (in 75–79 per cent of the cases), billing for individual lab tests performed as components of a single procedure (17 per cent), billing at higher than customary rates for home or office visits or specific services (13 per cent), billing for services rendered by a nonphysician (10 per cent), billing for services already paid for as part of a surgical or other procedure (3 per cent), and duplicate billing (2 per cent).

Pharmacy abuses included claims for greater than customary charges (51 per cent), claims for prescriptions not filled (33 per cent), and claims for prescriptions of greater quantity or price than actually dispensed (15 per cent). Labs were found to submit claims for services not rendered (45 per cent), for higher than customary rates (22 per cent) and for ineligible services (22 per cent).

Criticisms of the Massachusetts Medicaid program centered on data management: lack of a physician identification number, lack of a procedural code for lab services, the difficulty of identifying from lab records the physician ordering the test, failure to keep patient records up to date, and lack of summary data on service providers. Procedures to eliminate duplicate billing were suggested. The customary charge regulation for reimbursement was found "unclear, unadministrable and unenforceable." The requirement that telephone prescriptions be followed by written prescriptions was not being followed; this is the responsibility of the physician. Also, physicians must keep more complete and accurate records of prescriptions in order to allow for verification. Pharmacies should retain original prescriptions for 3 years instead of keeping only a log. Guidelines for action on reimbursement irregularities are proposed, including periodic review of the fee schedule for prescriptions.

References, 0. *Key words:* Drug utilization review.

SOCIAL AND REHABILITATION SERVICE. MEDICAL SERVICES ADMINISTRATION. Washington, D.C., Social and Rehabilitation Service, 1977.

1976

Revolution in Health Care

15

This symposium was organized by World Health Information Services, Inc. of New York and produced through an educational grant from Hoffmann-LaRoche, Inc.

Proceedings include abstracts and texts of papers and panel discussions on prepaid health care programs (including Health Maintenance Organizations), federal regulations on maximum allowable cost of prescription drugs (views pro and con), open and closed formulary programs (experiences in Mississippi and South Carolina), peer utilization and review (including the computer-assisted Peer Review Program developed by the San Joaquin Foundation for Medical Care and the Professional Standards Review Organization concept), and cooperation of public and private sectors in controlling health care costs.

References, 0. *Key words:* Drug utilization review, formularies, maximum allowable cost.

ANONYMOUS. Proceedings of a Symposium Held in Sacramento, California, September 8, 1975. Nutley, New Jersey, Hoffmann-LaRoche, Incorporated, 1976.

Social and Economic Aspects of Drug Utilization Research

46

Contains abstracts of federally-funded research reports and of the published literature, for 1960–1975, in 10 major research categories; each category includes a state-of-the-art report. The categories are: drug education research, pharmaceutical economics research, drug information research, pharmacy practice research, drug utilization research, drug insurance research, drug distribution research, pharmaceutical manpower research, drug surveillance research, and drug formulary system research. Includes an index to authors and project directors.

References, 0. *Key words:* Drug utilization review, formularies, reimbursement.

CONLEY, BERNARD E. Hamilton, Illinois, Drug Intelligence Publications, 1976.

Price Variations for Prescription Drugs

48

A price survey of two samples of prescription drugs was conducted in December 1973 in New York City, where in-store price posting was required and price advertising of prescription drugs forbidden, to investigate price competition and potential consumer gains from advertising. One sample consisted of 10 top drugs on the Master Drug List of prescription drugs used by the elderly; the second list of 10 drugs (with 4 overlapping) accounted for 81.5 per cent of the prescription drug component of the Consumers Price Index. The pharmacies were 3 chain and 3 independent stores in a Queens neighborhood. Price indexes ranging from 120.60 to 407.71 for sample 1 and 138.34 to 407.71 for sample 2, with medians of 146.39 and 201.30 respectively, indicate large potential savings for comparison shoppers. Coefficients of variation ranged from 8.45 per cent to 63.82 per cent in sample 1 and 11.59 per cent to 63.82 per cent in sample 2.

Since lower prices are more significant to the elderly, smaller sample 1 variations are in accord with Stigler's theory that a major source of price dispersion is lack of search by buyers. Average prices were lower in chain stores, by 20 per cent in sample 1 and 32 per cent in sample 2. Analysis of variance indicated a significant difference between store types, which can be attributed to the economics of large-scale operation. However, there was considerable variation by individual store and drug. Chains had lower market basket prices, but the difference was insignificant because of wide variations. Extrapolation to 1973 United States prescription costs of the 28 per cent difference between market baskets based on average and lowest store prices suggests a potential consumer saving of $1,337 million from increased price information. Price advertising would affect both buyer search and seller competition. Even if price differences partially reflect variations in services, the consumer would gain increased right to choose. It can be concluded that price posting does not necessarily reduce price variations.

Note: It is not clear to the abstractor why the statement of a lack of significance between store types is followed (p. 22) by a statement that this reinforces the importance of store type as the major factor in price differences.

References, 18.

DARDIS, RACHEL; and DOWDELL, D. *Journal of Retailing* 52 (3):15–26, Fall 1976.

Bibliography of Theses and Dissertations Relevant to Pharmacy Administration. 1970–1974

80

Annotations of approximately 700 masters theses and doctoral dissertations for 1970–1974 on topics in pharmacy administration are arranged in 9 major subject categories: pharmacy and pharmacists, pharmaceutical education, drugs, pharmaceutical industry, wholesaling, retail pharmacy operations, hospital pharmacy, history and law. More specific topics include drug payment systems, drug marketing and promotion, and prescription pricing in retail pharmacies and in hospitals. Theses and dissertations in 5 related areas are also included: health, administrative sciences, social sciences and humanities, the chemical industry and education. Author and title indexes are provided along with complete bibliographic information and University Microfilm number. Doctoral dissertation citations were obtained from *Dissertation Abstracts;* masters thesis citations were obtained from surveys of schools that have graduate programs in pharmacy administration.

References, 0.

See abstract 126, p. 46.

GARNER, DEWEY D., EDITOR. Bethesda, Maryland, American Association of Colleges of Pharmacy, 1976.

Dispensing Patterns under Third Party Programs

124

This paper compares the rank order of the most frequently prescribed drugs in a number of different third party programs with the *Pharmacy Times* listing of the top 200 drugs in the country. Specific differences are pointed out and it is concluded that the type of patient covered by the program, the presence or absence of a cost sharing arrangement and the degree of prescribing restrictions, i.e., a formulary, affect the position of specific drug products in the most-frequently-prescribed list.

Programs examined include private commercial insurance plans in the west and east, Medicaid programs both with and without a copayment, and a Medicaid program and a prepaid health plan with restrictive formularies. Drug manufacturers are encouraged to: (1) recognize the objectives of specific third party programs, (2) study the drug use of the programs with specific reference to the variables and restrictions imposed by the third party, and (3) provide information to program administrators in line with the plans, objectives and restrictions.

References, 0. *Key words:* Drug utilization review, formularies.

KENNARD, LON H.; and RODEN, DONALD R. *Medical Marketing and Media 11* (5):44, 46–47, 50–51, May 1976.

Comparative Approaches to Cost Constraints in Pharmaceutical Benefits Programs

141

Lee discusses United States and European approaches to constraints on drug expenditures under public health programs. He suggests that third-party programs reinforce the physician's tendency to use high-cost treatment options; for example, if only inpatient drugs are covered, the physician concerned with the patient's economic welfare will recommend hospitalization. It is illogical for public programs to encourage this kind of activity. Rising drug costs are due to world-wide increases in costs of raw materials and labor. Productivity may be hampered by the time and expenditures required to meet federal regulations.

He presents European experiences in determining utilization and controlling drug use by patient cost-sharing. Some countries exempt certain categories (for example, retirees) from copayment. He concludes that research and development must be encouraged and that each country's goals must include the optimization of quality and quantity of health care within available economic resources. He prefers constraints that will reinforce the competitive market system rather than those that involve coercion.

In a critique of Lee's remarks, Leif Schaumann suggests equitable distribution and accessibility of health care services as a national goal. He discusses the experience of the Scandinavian countries and the reliance on efficient centralized planning, and questions the usefulness of international expenditure comparisons because of problems of definition. He recommends limited price controls on retailers and concludes that because of the societal characteristics of the United States, pharmaceutical benefits are best expanded on a piecemeal basis to minimize economic, social, scientific and political consequences, and that foreign experiences have limited applicability to the United States.

T. Donald Rucker disputes Lee's explanation of drug industry pricing practices and suggests more careful consideration of overhead costs and price competition. He recommends the establishment of a national computerized drug record system to collect and analyze data on prescriptions initiated and dispensed. He questions the ability of market forces to effectively regulate drug prices. Government policy should include the cooperative development of a uniform cost accounting system.

References, not counted; footnotes used. *Key words:* Drug utilization review, patient cost sharing.

LEE, ARMISTEAD M. *In* Mitchell, Samuel A. and Link, Emery A., Editors. *Impact of Public Policy on Drug Innovation and Pricing.* Proceedings of the Third Seminar on Pharmaceutical Public Policy Issues, December 1975. Washington, D.C., American University, 1976. Pages 115–170, 170–177, 177–189.

Pharmaceutical Benefits under State Medical Assistance Programs

164

An annual compilation of data on state medical assistance drug programs. For each state, the following data are provided: (1) benefits provided and groups eligible, (2) expenditures for drugs by fiscal year, (3) how program is administered, (4) provisions relating to prescribed drugs, including general exclusions, formulary, prescribing or dispensing limitations and prescription charge formula, (5) miscellaneous remarks, (6) officials, consultants and committees, and (7) executive directors of state medical and pharmaceutical associations. An introductory portion provides selected background information as well as the names of HEW regional office officials, regional pharmacy consultants, and state Medicaid drug program administrators. Several charts are provided summarizing state data on total vendor payments for prescribed drugs, payments for prescribed drugs by category of aid, medical vendor payments by type of service, percentages of medical vendor payment by type of service, and Medicaid services state by state.

References, 0. *Key words:* Formularies, patient cost sharing, reimbursement.

NATIONAL PHARMACEUTICAL COUNCIL. Washington, D.C., The Council, 1976.

Prescription Drug Industry Factbook '76

178

A reference guide on the social and economic aspects of manufacturing and distributing prescription drugs, medical devices, and diagnostic equipment and materials. Discusses innovation, quality assurance (including problems of equivalence and bioavailability), sales and growth, the industry structure, employment and productivity, inflation and prescription prices, internal operations, the health care industry, medical devices and diagnostic products. Public third-party payments for drugs have risen 106.6 per cent from 1970 to 1975. Public third-party health care payments accounted for 39.7 per cent of all personal health expenditures in 1975, 21.7 per cent in 1960. Drugs and drug sundries accounted for 8.9 per cent of total health care expenditures in fiscal 1975. The average prescription price was $4.64 in 1975, $3.22 in 1960.

References, not counted; footnotes used.

PHARMACEUTICAL MANUFACTURERS ASSOCIATION. Washington, D.C.: The Association, 1976.

National Health Insurance and Prescription Benefits

195

Drug benefits in two legislative proposals for national health insurance are described; and possible roles for the pharmacist in helping to determine rational prescribing and pricing policies are considered.

A drug benefit program for ambulatory patients is difficult to administer because of the sheer volume of claims (although they involve only about 7 per cent of the personal health care budget), the various participants (manufacturers, wholesalers, physicians, pharmacists, patients) and inconsistencies in drug pricing, prescribing, dispensing and use.

The bill proposed by Senator Long provides drug coverage only for certain mental health outpatients who satisfy income eligibility requirements. The bill proposed by Senator Kennedy provides broad drug benefits for patients who receive medical services in organized settings, such as Health Maintenance Organizations, hospitals and clinics, but benefits are limited to those drugs considered appropriate for certain selected diseases. Both bills reflect concern about rational prescribing and use of drugs, and about socio-economic implications of drug pricing practices. Pharmacists may choose to adjust to the regulations resulting from enactment of national health insurance legislation, or may react more aggressively and provide leadership in dealing with the issues, for example, through improved accounting systems and better patient medication record keeping (the latter possibly through the use of a computerized patient ID system, so that complete patient records may be collated regardless of the number of pharmacies with which a patient deals).

References, 7. *Key words:* Drug utilization review, reimbursement.

RUCKER, T. DONALD. *Drug Intelligence and Clinical Pharmacy 10* (9):529–533, September 1976.

Innovation in the Pharmaceutical Industry

208 Presents an economic analysis of the drug industry, especially the costs of pharmaceutical research, examines empirical evidence and offers recommendations. Contains chapters on methodology, basic research and invention, characteristics of drug research, importance of industrial sources of new drugs, research activity and the size of the firm, competition by innovation, expected rate of return on pharmaceutical research and development, life of drug patents, promotional expenditures, quality of drugs and generic prescribing, price competition, the economic literature, and government and alternative goals for public policy. Reports that a large proportion of prescriptions for multi-source drugs are generic; since pharmacists can and do dispense multi-source prescriptions with low-priced drugs (whether written for brand or generic name), price competition is encouraged. Such substitution is surprisingly large, even though illegal in most states. Evaluates effectiveness of the FDA and the National Center for Drug Analysis. Discusses Maximum Allowable Cost regulations, expected to reduce the costs of drugs to the government, plus proposed legislation on formularies, generic drugs and patent rights. Appendix deals briefly with controversies on drug choice in hypertension, schizophrenia, and diabetes.

References, not counted; footnotes used. *Key words:* Formularies, maximum allowable cost, patents and prices.

SCHWARTZMAN, DAVID. Baltimore, Johns Hopkins University Press, 1976.

1975

A Comparison of Maintenance and Nonmaintenance Outpatient Prescription Directions, Durations of Coverage and Costs Per Day

75

Recent interest in Medicare coverage of outpatient prescriptions prompted a study to compare present economics and prescribing patterns for uninsured maintenance and nonmaintenance drug prescriptions.

Findings of the Task Force on Prescription Drugs and another report that maintenance drug prescription prices are higher indicated the need for detailed investigation of average cost per day, dosage directions (dosage), frequency of administration (frequency), quantity prescribed and dispensed (quantity) and length of therapy (duration). Data were collected in 1971 from 810 maintenance and 810 nonmaintenance prescriptions in 17 diverse pharmacies in a midwestern metropolitan area. One-way analysis of variance and analysis of covariance revealed that average quantity, price and duration are significantly higher for maintenance drugs. Dosages, frequencies and cost per day (even with quantities and frequencies controlled) are significantly lower.

Multiple linear regression analysis indicated that quantity and frequency were the most significant variables in duration and, in reverse order, in cost per day for users of maintenance drugs. Possible explanations for the finding that patients on maintenance drug therapy fare better economically ($.15 per day versus $.61 per day for nonmaintenance drug users, with prescription duration (without refills) averaging 53.6 days for the former and 12.1 days for the latter) are that frequent use of nonmaintenance drugs for acute conditions results in higher average frequency of administration; physicians may consider intervals between visits, potential discounts on large quantities and adequate supply for chronic illnesses in prescribing higher average quantities of maintenance drugs; and pharmacy costs per unit for nonmaintenance drugs like antibiotics may be higher or receive different gross margins.

There must be further investigation into the factors which influence physician choice of frequency and quantity on a maintenance drug prescription. More research into all factors involved is needed before a maintenance drug prescription benefit is added to Medicare.

References, 8. *Key words:* Drug utilization review.

GAGNON, JEAN P.; NELSON, ARTHUR A.; and RODOWSKAS, CHRISTOPHER A., JR. *Medical Care 13* (*1*):47–58, January 1975.

Drugs

94

Third-parties paid for 40.5 per cent of all personal health expenditures in 1970. Coverage ranged from 86.5 per cent for hospital care to 11.1 per cent for drugs and sundries. The 1.4 billion prescriptions purchased cost $4 billion. While per capita expenditures were $19.62, people over 65 averaged $50.94. Other variables included sex, race and place of residence. Most third-party programs pay the drug provider, usually with a deductible provision. The

Government Accounting Office criticized a drug interest-sponsored study that proposed basing reimbursement on usual and customary charges modified by a pharmacy "prescription service index" on the grounds that actual regional differences in operating costs do not warrant the variances recommended in state pricing formulas. The expected increase in third-party coverage for outpatient drugs requires better methods of discriminating on the basis of quality and cost differences.

The Puget Sound, Washington Group Health Cooperative, seems to be having success with an experimental drug insurance program. The HEW Task Force on Prescription Drugs urged coverage of outpatient prescriptions by the hospital component of Medicare, but recommended against a comprehensive program that would have cost $1.5 billion in 1971. It favored holding expenditures to some half million dollars by restricting coverage to long-term maintenance drugs, requiring coinsurance and imposing various administrative limitations such as maximum prescription quantities. The Task Force considered methods for determining drug acquisition costs and recommended reimbursing for the least expensive generally available chemical equivalent of acceptable quality. Effective price review mechanisms are important because of marked price differentials resulting from a lack of competitive conditions. A drug may be 40 times more expensive in Atlanta than New York, and low-income groups may pay much more than the affluent. Though government programs have been much slower than hospitals to turn to formularies as cost utilization control mechanisms, the HEW Task Force strongly favors their use. It remarked on the general professional acceptance and few problems in those countries that have used expert committees to design formularies.

References, 34. *Key words:* Formularies, maximum allowable cost, reimbursement, patient cost sharing.

HARRIS, SEYMOUR E. *In* Harris, Seymour E. *The Economics of Health Care. Finance and Delivery.* Berkeley, California, McCutchan Publishing Corporation, 1975. Pages 255–263.

Review of Literature on the Factors Affecting Drug Prescribing

98

This literature review enumerates the various factors affecting drug prescribing in Western countries. The influence of education on drug prescribing is difficult to establish, because the success of education varies from country to country. The effect of advertising on drug prescribing is questionable. While some say there is little effect, the drug industry continues to pour a sizeable percentage of sales revenue into drug promotion. The role of colleagues in spreading knowledge for prescribing is an important one, although their effect seems to be secondary to factors such as education and advertising. The factors of control and regulations measures involving official drug registration is narrowly used by health authorities, but studies indicate that such measures exert a positive effect if used effectively. Demands from society and patients, as well as doctor's characteristics, are two other factors mentioned; however, indications are that knowledge about the factors affecting prescribing is limited. National studies are necessary, since the nature of these factors may vary from one country to another. However, from the available literature, it appears that drug firms may be a major factor in Western countries. Further study is suggested to see whether it is more effective to control the prescription habits of the physician, or the factors affecting him, such as advertising. Other factors, too, need further analysis.

References, 72. *Key words:* Drug utilization review.

HEMMINKI, ELINA. *Social Science and Medicine* 9 (2):111–116, February 1975.

A Commentary on "The Interdependence of Prescription Drugs and other Health Care Costs": Some Implications for Research

103

Dr. Hornbrook, an economist with the National Center for Health Services Research of HEW, responds to an earlier article by Mr. Armistead Lee of the Pharmaceutical Manufacturers Association. The debate is concerned with the economics of the drug industry and its market, and deals with adverse drug reactions, insurance coverage for inpatient and outpatient drugs and other medical care goods and services, inflation and price competition in the drug industry, drug product proliferation and promotional activities, and other aspects of costs, profits and prices.

Dr. Hornbrook calls for the continued investigation of these problems through appropriately designed research studies, the formulation of operational definitions, and the analysis and consideration of all viewpoints before formulating policies to control drug costs. For example, research on the costs of adverse drug reactions (ADRs) requires the specification of the purpose of the analysis, the definition of an ADR and the definition of relevant costs. Does an ADR include any "unexpected" reactions to a particular drug, or does it include all undesired side effects, predicted or not? Does the cost of an ADR include patient suffering and lost productivity as well as treatment expenditures? Other policy issues requiring analysis include: uneven insurance coverage of different medical care goods and services; limited coverage of outpatient drugs as a financial barrier to filling prescriptions, thus affecting treatment of medical problems; physician attitudes toward drug substitution; actual acquisition costs to pharmacists; product proliferation and price competition; and the Maximum Allowable Cost program.

References, 10.

See abstracts 143, page 25; 144, page 26.

HORNBROOK, MARK C. *Drugs in Health Care* 2 (4):255–261, Fall 1975.

The Interdependence of Prescription Drugs and other Health Care Costs

143

Discussed here are several of the misconceptions about the economic structure of the drug industry and market. The drug portion of health care costs has been the one with the least inflation, and although the price index for drugs rose in 1974, the actual cost of the drug to the consumer has been cut by 50 per cent since 1960. This is due to the fact that per capita personal income is twice that in 1960. It is important in a health care program to optimize the use of the least expensive factor, in this case drug therapy, in order to keep costs down, but the provision of quality care must also be a priority. Many are concerned with "product proliferation," where multiple versions or variations of a drug result in price or therapeutic competition. However, the social benefits accrued from this override the costs involved.

Research-based pharmaceutical manufacturers have high marketing expenditures, necessary in order to introduce new products to the market and to provide information for physicians concerning the availability and proper use of drugs. The ratio of promotion to sales has declined, but advertising expenditures have increased and, thus, do not reflect the cutback. Although the average rate of return on investment is higher in the drug industry, this rate is often overstated for companies with large investments in advertising and research and development. Under the Maximum Allowable Cost (MAC) program of HEW, the savings that have been projected in government reimbursement are exaggerated and it seems likely that administrative costs exceed these savings. Effective utilization of drug prescribing and increased physician awareness of drug information would better reduce the rate of drug expenditures than would imposing constraints only on one aspect (drug therapy) of the overall health care program.

References, 15. *Key words:* Drug utilization review, maximum allowable cost.

See abstracts 103, page 25; 144, page 26.

LEE, ARMISTEAD M. *Drugs in Health Care* 2 (2):75–85, Spring 1975.

A Reply to Hornbrook

144

Mr. Lee, of the Pharmaceutical Manufacturers Association, replies to an earlier article by Dr. Mark Hornbrook, an economist with the National Center for Health Services Research of HEW, in which Dr. Hornbrook was commenting on an earlier article by Mr. Lee entitled "The Interdependence of Prescription Drugs and Other Health Care Costs." Mr. Lee states that he is primarily concerned with drug costs relative to other health care costs, while Dr. Hornbrook seems concerned with drug prices and the performance of the pharmaceutical industry. There is controversy about competitive conditions and the relationship between costs and benefits, and agreement that more data are needed on these issues. Mr. Lee maintains that the extent and cost of adverse drug reactions has been exaggerated; that hospitalization costs must be considered in cases where patients are hospitalized in order to receive drugs covered by insurance plans; that drugs are the least inflationary component of health care expenditures; that research and development expenditures as well as manufacturing and marketing costs must be considered in drug pricing; and that product proliferation and competition have a net social benefit. The Pharmaceutical Manufacturers Association favors drug research legislation and more rigid enforcement of FDA regulations.

References, 0.

See abstracts 143, page 25; 103, page 25.

LEE, ARMISTEAD M. *Drugs in Health Care* 2 (4):261–265, Fall 1975.

Review of Victor I. Fuchs, "Who Shall Live?"

200

The book reviewed—subtitled "health, economics and social choice"—focuses on three health care components: physicians, hospitals and drugs. Problems in health care provision and factors affecting payment are discussed. Recommendations are made for the development of an effective national health policy. A noteworthy section deals with catastrophic insurance and "caring" versus "curing" forms of treatment, questioning governmental obligation for the former. Also, the effect of personal behavior—driving, smoking, drinking—on the utilization of health insurance benefits is examined. Prospective budgeting, based on average costs and the capitation method of payment, is discussed in relation to prescription drug price control. The chapter on drugs is criticized for implying a high correlation between drug use and ultimate health status, leading the author to support more relaxed standards for certifying new products. Coordination of drug use (possibly by computer-maintained prescription profiles) is suggested by the reviewer as an alternative to the author's recommendation that any one patient receive all drugs from a single pharmacist. Reducing pharmaceutical prices on large quantity sales is justified in traditional economic terms; again, the reviewer disagrees. In sum, the Fuchs book constitutes a substantial contribution to the literature on the functioning of the health care system in the United States.

References, 0.

See abstract 71, page 28.

RUCKER, T. DONALD. *Drugs in Health Care* 2 (4):266–268, Fall 1975.

Role of the Pharmaceutical Industry in a Dynamic Health Care System

202

Trends in health care delivery and financing, and their potential influence on drug industry practices and controls, are discussed. These include quality control mechanisms (such as Professional Standards Review Organizations), prevention programs, efficient use of health care resources, economically sound reimbursement policies, patient sophistication, and the implementation of a comprehensive national health insurance plan.

Drug benefits under national health insurance require processing costs of approximately $2.00 per unit. To reduce this amount to an acceptable level (approximately 25¢), copayment programs and computerized record keeping are necessary. A formulary will help control costs by excluding drug benefits from products with no or marginal therapeutic value. Also, promotional activities of drug suppliers could be restricted to help minimize unneeded prescribing. Some uncovered prescriptions, however, will be paid for by patients directly or through supplemental private coverage.

Drug utilization under insurance programs is expected to increase (approximately 10–15 per cent), at least during the early years, because of larger prescription orders and the encouragement of untreated persons to seek medical care (usually for conditions amenable to drug therapy). Producer costs are discussed in terms of a model distribution system, professional education, research and development expenditures, patent and marketing rights, and corporate profits.

References, 13. *Key words:* Formularies, patient cost sharing.

RUCKER, T. DONALD. *Drugs in Health Care* 2 (2):86–95, Spring 1975.

Drugs in Nursing Homes: Misuse, High Costs, and Kickbacks

249 Analyzes drug distribution in 23,000 United States nursing homes (1959–1974) and gives examples and testimony supporting lax controls and the unfortunate consequences for both the nursing home patient and the American taxpayer.

Drug distribution in nursing homes is inefficient and ineffective. Physicians are rarely in attendance and nurses are overworked, so too often the responsibility for administering medication falls to aides and orderlies who have had little training. Nursing homes are the most likely places for adverse drug reactions and 20–40 per cent of drugs administered are in error. Patients are frequently tranquilized to keep them quiet; tranquilizers constitute almost 20 per cent of all drugs administered in nursing homes. Kickbacks from the pharmacy to the nursing home operator for the privilege of filling nursing home prescriptions amount to approximately 25 per cent of total prescription charges. This is aggravated when public reimbursement programs such as Medicaid/Medicare allow the nursing home to act as a "middle man" between the pharmacy and the source of payment. Public Law 92-603 (November 1972) prohibits kickbacks but HEW has never published regulations to implement or enforce the law. Recommends periodic medical review of long-term care facilities and treatment.

References, 0.

UNITED STATES SENATE. SPECIAL COMMITTEE ON AGING. Subcommittee on Long-Term Care. Nursing Home Care in the United States: Failure in Public Policy. Supporting Paper No. 2. Ninety-fourth Congress. First Session. Washington, D.C., U.S. Government Printing Office, 1975.

1974

Drugs

71 Drug expenditures account for 10 per cent of total health expenditures; however, several aspects of this industry are unique and warrant examination. Only 40 per cent of the industry's dollar is spent for production. An excess (when compared to other industries) is allocated to advertising and marketing. Drug prices could be substantially reduced if these areas were de-emphasized. The same point is made against the industry's profit, which is also more (percentagewise) than other industries. Economic arguments are presented supporting generic prescribing, furthered by the American Pharmaceutical Association. The Pharmaceutical Manufacturers Association develops a rebuttal on the grounds that physician control of the patient is necessary for optimum patient care. The savings from generic prescribing are going to increase, as many popular drugs are shortly coming off patents.

References, 0. *Key words:* substitution.

See abstract 200, page 27.

FUCHS, VICTOR R. *In* Fuchs, Victor R. *Who Shall Live?* New York, Basic Books, 1974. Pages 120–124.

National Prescription Audit. General Information Report

107

The National Prescription Audit, a nationwide market survey, includes volume and price data on total prescriptions, generic prescriptions and new pharmaceutical products, presented in 26 tables. Generic products accounted for 10.6 per cent of all new prescriptions in 1974. The average retail price in 1974 for a new prescription was $4.70, up from $2.17 in 1952. The average retail price for a generic prescription was $3.75. Ten drug manufacturers account for more than 50 per cent of all new prescriptions. Additional tables show consumer expenditures for new and refill prescriptions, average retail prices for new prescriptions in 10 therapeutic categories, and average retail prices for new prescriptions of 20 frequently prescribed generic products.

References, 0.

IMS AMERICA. Ambler, Pennsylvania, IMS America, Limited, 1974.

Drug Benefits in Health Insurance

160

In the United States, drug benefits are becoming an integral element of health insurance plans. By 1971, more than half of the population carried some type of drug coverage, about 80 per cent of which was provided for under major medical insurance policies. The basic features of several plans in effect both in Canada and the United States are outlined and evaluated according to their administration, methods of reimbursement, cost control and distribution. Distribution is effected through contractual agreement with participating pharmacies, pharmacy associations, plan-owned pharmacies, or mail-order drug services like those offered by Health Insurance Program. Attempts to evaluate and improve utilization are somewhat hampered by the variation among those complying with the existing rules. Methods employed to control utilization include copayment, emphasis on generic prescribing, limiting quantities and refills, and encouraging the physician to prescribe less frequently and profusely. There is some discussion of provisions for drug benefits in a design for a national health insurance scheme.

References, 30. *Key words:* Other countries, patient cost sharing, substitution.

MULLER, CHARLOTTE. *International Journal of Health Services* 4 (1):157–170, Winter 1974.

Prescribing Patterns in the New York City Medicaid Program

187 A sample of 5,271 prescription orders for both prescription and over-the-counter (OTC) drugs submitted to the New York City Medicaid program was analyzed by therapeutic category. The cost of medication by category and the frequency of generic prescriptions by category was determined.

The sample consisted of prescriptions on every fifth invoice submitted on May 20, 1971. Drugs prescribed were categorized into sixteen therapeutic classes according to the formulary of the American Society of Hospital Pharmacists. The most frequently prescribed classes of drugs were central nervous system drugs (21.1 per cent), systemic anti-infectives (15.7 per cent) and antihistamines (8.1 per cent). The physician has the option under the Medicaid program to prescribe by generic name or by brand name. Among prescription drugs, generic prescribing was most frequent for cardiovascular drugs (41 per cent), anti-infectives (23 per cent) and spasmolytic agents (18 per cent). Great variation in the frequency of generic prescribing existed among the subcategories of each drug category. Overall, an average of 13 per cent of drug orders for prescription drugs were written by generic name. Generic prescriptions for OTC drugs were for single or multiple vitamin products.

Comparison with prescribing patterns found in other studies revealed no significant differences for most categories. Specific areas of difference could be explained by the nature of health care services for the New York City Medicaid population. Cost analysis of the sample prescription orders indicated the average price of prescription drugs was $4.24 and of OTC drugs $2.06, for an average of $3.79 for all medications. This compares favorably with the "average prescription price" (unspecified as to prescription or OTC medications) of $3.92 determined in a 1971 survey by *American Druggist.* The paper concludes with a general discussion on cost-savings due to generic prescribing.

References, 17. *Key words:* Drug utilization review.

ROSENBERG, STEPHEN N.; BERENSON, LOUISE B.; KAVALER, FLORENCE; and GORELIK, ELIHU A. *Medical Care 12* (2):138–151, February 1974.

Drug Use. Data, Sources, and Limitations

192 A national drug information system clearing house is described as a means of ensuring the privacy of patient-care considerations over economic considerations in the implementation of national health insurance. The system would record and retrieve data for clinical, administrative, educational and research needs relating to drug use, and be compatible with a future general health care information network. Pharmacists would record prescriptions dispensed on terminals and the information would be transmitted to regional computer centers for analysis and storage (the clearing houses). In the future, terminals could be placed in physicians' offices for more direct transmission of prescription orders (to be retrieved and dispensed by pharmacists). Clearing houses would develop drug and patient profiles and would transmit third-party insurance claims. Professional access to data would be free of time constraints. In one proposed system, clinicians could conduct a concurrent review of prescription options and problems while the patient was being treated.

Costs of a national drug information network are estimated at "well under" $600 million annually; expected annual savings exceed $4 billion. One risk is the likelihood that third-party interests, and not patient and professional needs, would govern system and operation. Sources of data for the information system include the United States Bureau of Census and the Pharmaceutical Manufacturers Association (production data), the National Center for Health Statistics and Social Security Administration (data on drug use) and studies conducted by organizations such as the National Institute of Mental Health. However, much information is out of date or unavailable. The acquisition of comprehensive and current prescription information is vital to support patient care, therefore a national information system should be considered.

References, 24.

See abstract 142, page 187.

RUCKER, T. DONALD. *Journal of the American Medical Association 230* (6):888–890, November 11, 1974.

Public Policy Considerations in the Pricing of Prescription Drugs in the United States

198

The United States spent about $10 billion for prescribed drugs in 1973, and government insurance programs paid for over 27 per cent of this. Other justifications for government interest in drug pricing are the consumer's relative subservience to his illness, the pharmaceutical marketplace and professional expertise; the presumed high social utility of federal legend products; and the responsibility increasingly delegated to third-party insurers.

There are several inadequately discussed problems in the relationship of product pricing to actual cost. 1969 data for 9 important pharmaceuticals, which are probably still roughly valid, show that a median of only 9 per cent of wholesale prices represented direct expenses. Standard trade costs from the *Red Book* indicate that active ingredient amounts frequently do not correlate with prices. The relationship between size of package and price is similarly unpredictable.

Another questionable practice is differentiation in price by type of buyer without regard to quantities purchased. The biggest dispensing price problem is how to relate prescription charges to true overhead costs. Studies in several states show a very haphazard relationship now. A uniform cost-accounting system is the obvious solution. Other issues to be settled are an appropriate level of profit, for which a good cost-accounting system is prerequisite, and the role of incentives when both legitimate commercial and professional interests are involved.

Problems with prescription price posting—its promotional aspects, relative lack of effect on product cost and operational defects—can be minimized by adoption of a 1972 California Pharmaceutical Association proposal that pharmacies simply post a flat overhead fee to be applied to all prescriptions. Listing the dispensing services involved would further enhance consumer understanding. Third-party programs play a major role in obscuring economic relationships that should be reflected in prescription prices by reimbursing without regard to actual operating expenses or level of professional services. Failure to rationalize pricing mechanisms before a national health insurance program would bring imposed solutions.

References, 5.

RUCKER, T. DONALD. *International Journal of Health Services* 4 (*1*):171–179, Winter 1974.

Review of Pharmaceutical Manufacturers Association, "Pharmaceutical Payment Programs—an Overview"

199 The work under consideration—a contribution to the prescription drug insurance literature from the Pharmaceutical Manufacturers Association—treats current issues such as the following: Health Maintenance Organizations, Medicaid drug programs, techniques for administering drug insurance programs (including computer claims processing), the probability of national health insurance, the growth of private health insurance, prescription drug utilization and costs, third-party coverage of pharmaceutical services, and outpatient drug benefits under various existing and proposed health insurance schemes. The report attempts to offer differing viewpoints on these issues.

The report can be criticized for the following: being somewhat dated and thus omitting important information on current research and legislation; unclear data in some charts and tables and some unclear or incorrect terminology in the report and in the glossary; failing to note that many drug products are patented and therefore unlikely to be affected by market forces or by the HEW Maximum Allowable Cost (MAC) program; and failing to discuss the role of competition in drug pricing.

Appendices offer useful descriptive data on HMO legislation, national health insurance proposals, drug payment plans, and prescription insurance carriers.

References, 0.

See abstract 177, page 35.

RUCKER, T. DONALD. *Drugs in Health Care 1* (*1*):52–54, Summer 1974.

Pills, Profits, and Politics

216 This book examines various aspects of drug products and their manufacture, drug promotion, drug safety, efficacy and quality, drug prices, pharmacy, OTC's, government research support and drug regulation, government drug purchases (for the military, Veterans Administration, Public Health Service, Medicare/Medicaid), adverse reactions, rational prescribing and future goals. Tables on drug industry sales, profits, recalls, wholesale and retail prices of prescription and OTC drugs, per capita health expenditures and advertising volume are presented. The chapter on drug quality and generic prescribing (pp. 138–170) discusses the 1967 Nelson hearings on the drug industry and the HEW Task Force on Prescription Drugs. The problems of determining generic, chemical, biological and clinical equivalents are analyzed and anti-substitution laws are discussed. The chapter on drug prices (pp. 171–189) discusses prices in community pharmacies, hospitals, nursing homes and for government agencies (data 1970 or earlier). Ways of increasing the efficiency of pharmacy operations and reducing drug costs, comparison shopping, limiting promotional activities of drug manufacturers, and making use of a little-known federal law to override the patent law and have drugs manufactured at lower prices for government purchase (for example, in the Medicare program) are also discussed.

References, Forty-four pages of notes and references. *Key words:* Drug utilization review, formularies, patents and prices, reimbursement, substitution.

SILVERMAN, MILTON; and LEE, PHILIP R. Berkeley, University of California Press, 1974.

Effects of a Medicaid Program on Prescription Drug Availability and Acquisition

226

A random sample of 241 welfare recipients in a small Mississippi community with two pharmacies was studied, by interviews and prescription audits, both before (April 1–June 30, 1970) and after (April 1–June 30, 1971) the initiation of Medicaid, to determine drug availability and utilization. Records of prescriptions dispensed (new and refill) to the patients for the pre-Medicaid period were collected from the two pharmacies; post-Medicaid data were made available by printout from the Mississippi Medicaid Commission. Also, for comparative purposes, data on all new prescriptions for the two time periods were collected from 10 pharmacies in another part of the state.

Patients were divided into four groups: (1) no prescriptions filled before or after Medicaid; (2) prescriptions filled before but not after; (3) prescriptions filled after but not before; (4) prescriptions filled before and after. Twenty-five patients in each group were interviewed by a single trained interviewer. Eliminating persons seeing "dispensing" physicians (because of the difficulty in obtaining prescribing data), the results were as follows: Group (1) includes 43.8 per cent of the sample; (2) includes 12.4 per cent of the sample, 91 prescriptions received; (3) includes 17.8 per cent, 255 prescriptions received; (4) 25.9 per cent and 822 prescriptions received. Ninety-five and four-tenths per cent of the post-Medicaid prescriptions were dispensed at the 2 community pharmacies.

The difference in number of prescriptions dispensed before and after Medicaid was substantial and the average number of different drugs utilized per patient increased from 2.68 to 3.64. The average quantity of tablets or capsules dispensed per prescription (representing 76 per cent of all prescriptions dispensed and most of the maintenance drug therapy) increased from 45.00 to 48.35. The three-month average cost per patient increased from $18.96 to $42.54. The average price for all prescriptions rose from $3.58 to $4.49. Unit price data for the ten most frequently prescribed drugs are provided. The finding of differences between quantity dispensed and quantity prescribed (usually attributable to failure to obtain refills) has medical and economic implications; since further treatment will probably be required, additional expenses will be incurred. Although no formulary was used, it is suggested as a method not only to control costs, but also to encourage rational prescribing.

References, 9. *Key words:* Drug utilization review, formularies.

SMITH, MICKEY C.; and GARNER, DEWEY D. *Medical Care* 12 (7):571–581, July 1974.

1973

Source Options in HMO Pharmacy Service

16

Each Health Maintenance Organization (HMO) should develop a pharmacy component which best meets the needs of its community. Several methods are available to an HMO for the provision of pharmaceutical services: (1) to establish its own on-site pharmacy, (2) to establish an on-site pharmacy on a contract basis, (3) to utilize existing neighborhood pharmacies which would provide services to HMO patrons under direct contract with the HMO—"the vendor option," (4) to contract with an independent pharmaceutical services administration group which would take charge of the organization and the monitoring of existing pharmaceutical providers, and (5) a combination of the above options.

Several advantages and disadvantages of the vendor option are discussed. Some of its advantages are: (1) no expenditures are required by the HMO for personnel directly related to the acquisition, storage and distribution of drugs, (2) no expenditures relating to the maintenance of a drug inventory are required, (3) convenience for the user due to the close location of neighborhood pharmacies, and (4) patients tend to have more contact and will consult more often with a neighborhood pharmacist than with a pharmacist located in an on-site pharmacy. Some of the disadvantages of the vendor system are: (1) the cost involved in processing vendor reimbursement claims, and (2) the difficulty in monitoring and controlling the quality or cost of the vendor's services; the need to establish elaborate monitoring mechanisms.

One guide in choosing to establish an on-site pharmacy is that an HMO should serve at least 5,000 patients. Several methods to control the costs of an on-site pharmacy are: (1) careful purchasing control, (2) accurate determination of staffing needs and the proper utilization of the staff, and (3) careful planning of the design and location of the pharmacy and the use of efficient equipment.

References, 0. *Key words:* Direct provision, drug utilization review, reimbursement.

ANONYMOUS. *Hospitals* 47 (24):75–77, December 16, 1973.

Availability and Cost of Urinary Antibacterials in a Metropolitan Area

58

Since price may deter a patient from obtaining a prescription and specific prescription cost information is rarely available to physicians, nine pharmacies in the Chicago area were surveyed to determine the prices of the most frequently recommended drugs for treating bacterial infections of the urinary tract. Actual charges to private patients for three-week courses of average dosage were obtained in September to October 1972 from two chain drug stores, three independent pharmacies and four teaching hospital outpatient pharmacies. The authors had either worked in these stores or knew the pharmacists well enough to consider their quotations reliable. The establishments varied in location, though all but three hospital pharmacies served predominantly middle-class clienteles. The data gathered are presented in a table showing prices of corresponding trademark drugs under fifteen official names of nonproprietary drugs.

The findings include that penicillin G and tetracycline were the only substances generally stocked under nonproprietary labels. Sulfisoxazole, Mandelamine®, NegGram® and Keflex® were the only specialties stocked by all stores. The four hospital pharmacies stocked only one preparation of each drug, suggesting that the attending physicians and the pharmacy and therapeutics committees of their hospitals accept substitution. Suspensions and syrups were much more expensive than capsules or tablets of the same drug. Nonproprietary products were almost always much cheaper than trademarked analogs, but were seldom available. Price variations between different brands of the same drug in a given pharmacy were usually greater than variations between the same brand in different stores, where variations in administration and levels of service come into play. Cephalosporins are so expensive that they should be used only when penicillins or sulfonamides are contra-indicated or ineffective.

References, 14. *Key words:* Substitution.

ELLIS, ROBERT F.; and SICE, JEAN. *Journal of Chronic Diseases 26 (10)*:617–622, 1973.

Pharmaceutical Payment Programs—An Overview: The Financing of Prescription Medicines Through Third Party Programs

177

This review examines issues associated with third-party payment for prescription drugs and suggests ways of resolving the issues so that the public and the pharmaceutical industry will not be adversely affected in receiving and providing high quality health care services. Health care trends and the growth of private health insurance, the economics of prescription drug product supply and demand, current third-party prescription payment programs (Blue Cross, union programs and administrative services such as PAID Prescriptions, Inc.), and the present and potential impact on the pharmaceutical industry of Medicare/Medicaid, Health Maintenance Organization's (HMO) and national health insurance are discussed. The concept of a federal formulary and the types of drug benefits proposed by various national health insurance bills are reviewed. The overview concludes that if problems with prepayment and the negotiation of dispensing fees can be overcome, approximately 60 per cent of outpatient prescription drug costs will be covered by third-party programs by the 1980's. Appendices include HMO legislative proposals (1972–1973), national health insurance legislative proposals, pharmaceutical drug payment programs, prepaid prescription plans and a glossary.

References, 133. *Key words:* Formularies, reimbursement, substitution.

See abstract 199, page 32.

PHARMACEUTICAL MANUFACTURERS ASSOCIATION. Washington, D.C., The Association, 1973.

Economic Aspects of Drug Overuse

193 This attempt to analyze the economic ramifications of American drug overuse immediately encounters complex conceptual and methodological problems, even with a narrow interpretation of drugs as legend pharmaceuticals, over-the-counter products, or illicitly used substances. These three categories exceeded $13 billion in market sales in 1972, and their economic impact was much greater. Some factors that complicate the task of measuring and interpreting this impact are: (1) patterns of abuse change, (2) definitional rigidities make it difficult to study aggregate costs associated with an illness, (3) difficulty in obtaining national statistics on illicit drug use or segregating pharmaceutical costs and profits, (4) drug purchases not always synonymous with consumption, (5) wastefulness when a drug is marketed without concern for its ineffectiveness, but a legitimate expense when a drug is found to have unforeseeable dangerous side effects, (6) appraisal requiring established standards regarding drug utility and sound therapy, and (7) assumptions which must be made about what savings could be achieved by developing a more rational system of communicating drug information.

There are negative economic consequences when medical intervention is indicated but drug use is inappropriate. Examples are the use of hundreds of drugs later deemed "ineffective" and millions of dollars' worth of irrational combination products, or the large-scale prescribing of antibiotics for viral diseases. The costs of preventable deaths and institutional care resulting from adverse drug reactions are at least $4 billion a year. Professional interface with regional computerized drug data banks could control much of this waste for less than $1 billion a year. Other action is needed to get at problems of self-administration. Economic evaluation is more difficult when a medical problem is questionable or nonexistent. Even if the use of psychotropic agents to improve social functioning is accepted as legitimate, cheaper substitutes should be used and manufacturers' promotional efforts should be terminated. The more diffuse action of these agents may also mean a broader range of costs. The fiscal 1974 federal budget calls for nearly $720 million for drug abuse programs. This does not begin to measure the costs of state or interest group programs, meetings and legislative deliberations, etc., not to mention the long-term social costs. Additional considerations in trying to develop meaningful controls include the exclusion of ambulatory patients from drug insurance coverage, changes in personal attitudes about tolerating discomfort and the reluctance of drug specialists to promulgate and enforce standards. Finally, progress against drug abuse requires improving the nation's general quality of life.

References, 27.

RUCKER, T. DONALD. *Medical Annals of the District of Columbia* 42 (12):609–614, December 1973.

The Mail-Order Prescription Drug Industry

255 Six general features of the services of the mail-order prescription drug industry are discussed: patient characteristics, prescription pricing, prescription processing, prescription dispensing, prescription shipping, and prescription volume and drugs dispensed. The industry profile was compiled from a survey of ten of the largest mail-order prescription suppliers. These ten organizations, selected from a listing of the sixty known mail-order suppliers, are responsible for about 90 per cent of the total volume of mail-order prescription drugs (estimated at 17 million prescriptions annually) in the United States.

A standard set of questions was used in the survey, which was conducted through personal and telephone interviews. A few of the many specific characteristics of the services discussed are: (1) most mail-order suppliers serve elderly patients with chronic conditions, who use many drugs and who live in rural areas, (2) mail-order prices are generally competitive with drug prices in urban areas; some organizations offer a discount on prescription prices to their members, (3) firms generally take precautionary steps to screen out fraudulent orders, (4) most organizations do not maintain drug-use profiles of patients, nor perform drug interaction monitoring of patient's drug regimens and (5) drug dispensing operations are supervised by pharmacists.

Specific services offered by individual suppliers are discussed; for example, the Veterans Administration program is unique in that it is the only organization allowed by postal regulations to dispense narcotics through the mails. A discussion follows on two issues which are generally raised by opponents of the mail-order industry: the alleged disruption of the traditional physician-patient-pharmacist relationship, and the potential for fraud in prescription mail-orders. There is a lack of factual evidence to support or disprove these claims. The authors suggest that the economic competition of the mail-order suppliers may force retail pharmacists to oppose them. An objective evaluation of practices and the development of standards for the prescription mail-order industry is recommended.

References, 6.

WERTHEIMER, ALBERT, I.; and KNOBEN, JAMES E. *Health Services Reports 88* (9):852–856, November 1973.

1972

Two Controversial Problems in Third Party Outpatient Prescription Plans

78

In the mid sixties, insurance experts were predicting that outpatient prescription drug coverage would expand rapidly in the years to come. By 1970, however, only 15 per cent of outpatient prescription charges were paid for by third parties. The authors ascribe this slow growth to difficulties in four major areas: (1) the large number of small claims generated by drug coverage, (2) the high cost of processing each claim, (3) the high risk to insurance companies because of the widespread utilization of drugs, and (4) difficulties associated with reimbursing pharmacists for product cost and dispensing services. This article focuses specifically on the fourth problem area.

A brief chronology of the growth of private and public drug insurance is presented, followed by a more detailed analysis of the ingredient cost controversy and the professional fee controversy.

The major problem in determining ingredient cost is that different pharmacies pay different prices for drug products. Insurance companies and government programs took the position that they would reimburse actual acquisition cost. Pharmacists, on the other hand, argue for reimbursement based on average wholesale costs, which were estimated to be 10–15 per cent higher than actual acquisition costs. The authors suggest that a uniform cost for prescription drugs be set that is halfway between average wholesale and actual acquisition costs.

Insurance companies wish to avoid reimbursing for professional services on the basis of usual and customary charges because of auditing difficulties and the ease with which such charges may rise. Most plans chose to reimburse pharmacists on the basis of a fixed professional fee. These programs ran into legal difficulties in the 1960's however. In 1969, the Virginia Supreme Court ruled that the use of a fixed fee by Blue Cross was a "per se" violation of price fixing. Soon thereafter, the Illinois Supreme Court ruled the opposite in a similar case. Government programs are not bound by these decisions and the Medicaid program favors a fixed fee for reimbursement.

References, 18.

See abstract 65, page 157.

GAGNON, JEAN P.; and RODOWSKAS, CHRISTOPHER A., JR. *Journal of Risk and Insurance 39* (4):603–611, December 1972.

The United Auto Workers Negotiated Prepaid Prescription Drug Program

83

The success of the United Auto Workers (UAW) prepaid prescription drug program, initiated in 1969, has demonstrated the feasibility of a drug prepayment plan on a nationally uniform basis. The plan is primarily administered through a national Blue Cross-Blue Shield arrangement; commercial insurance carriers are used in a few regions of the nation. The Michigan Blue Cross-Blue Shield has responsibility for the administration of the plan. Participating private pharmacists are reimbursed on the basis of "acquisition cost plus a dispensing fee." The basic copayment per prescription is $2. Plan members can patronize a nonparticipating pharmacy, but will generally not be reimbursed 100 per cent (less the $2 copayment). The "problem" areas of the plan and possible future developments offered as solutions to these problems are explored. The three areas needing assessment are: (1) whether a fair price is being paid to the vendor and for the program, (2) whether only drugs which are needed are being prescribed, and (3) whether the program is being administered efficiently. Incentivies to the pharmacist to reduce drug costs and the possible establishment of a utilization review and audit control program are discussed.

References, 1. *Key words:* Drug utilization review.

GOLDBERG, THEODORE; and LOREN, EUGENE L. *Journal of the American Pharmaceutical Association NS12* (8):422–425, August 1972.

Controlling Drug Costs

162

Research indicating that drug costs could be reduced by substituting generic or similar items of frequently prescribed drugs suggests several ways of controlling drug expenditures. Data from a mid-Atlantic county of 112,000 people in 1968 showed aggregate savings of $34,709 by substituting similarly acting drugs, and $22,931 by substituting generic equivalents for some of the twenty most frequently prescribed drugs. Average prescription prices are presented for eleven drugs and their substitutes.

Thus, reducing costs on just a small number of widely prescribed drug products will result in considerable savings in a health insurance program. Other suggestions for reducing drug costs—and improving the quality of prescribing—include (1) standards for drug manufacturers such that physicians will be more willing to prescribe generic products, (2) shorter patent periods for drugs, (3) continuing education and relicensing programs, especially for older physicians, to assure appropriate prescribing, (4) withdrawal of worthless drugs and higher standards of effectiveness for the introduction of new drugs, (5) limiting health insurance coverage on products used without specific indication (for example, tranquilizers), and (6) formularies and utilization review programs.

References, 1. *Key words:* Drug utilization review, formularies.

MULLER, CHARLOTTE; STOLLEY, PAUL D.; and BECKER, MARSHALL H. *American Journal of Public Health 62* (*6*):755–756, June 1972.

Pharmacy Involvement in the Neighborhood Health Center Environment

184

The planning, development and implementation of a neighborhood health center pharmacy service in Tuscon, Arizona is described in detail. The service was developed by the University of Arizona College of Pharmacy.

The health center is located in a low-income area predominantly populated by Mexican-Americans. The administration of the health center is discussed. Planning for the pharmacy program was done in close cooperation with representatives of the community and with community pharmacists. The program involves a combination system of in-house and vendor pharmacy services. The in-house facility provides a full range of pharmaceutical services and maintains a patient data record for all medications prescribed and dispensed for each patient, regardless of whether the drug is obtained at the in-house Center pharmacy or at a vendor pharmacy. Guidelines for vendor pharmacies provide control over the quality and quantity of services offered, the cost of prescriptions, the items contained in the vendor's formulary and prescription renewal procedures.

Thirty-six of the seventy-six community pharmacies in Tuscon are vendor pharmacies. A Grievance Committee has been established to ensure good communication between the neighborhood health center pharmacy and the vendor pharmacies. All parties benefit educationally from the program: vendor pharmacists are required to attend programs instituted by the Center and students in the College of Pharmacy have the opportunity to obtain on-the-job experience while receiving college credit.

References, 6.

ROBLES, RAMON R.; and WINSHIP, HENRY W. III. *American Journal of Hospital Pharmacy 29* (*1*):68–71, January 1972.

Economic Problems in Drug Distribution

194 Evidence is presented to show the inefficient use of resources and services in the distribution of prescribed pharmaceuticals, resulting in serious economic difficulties. In 1971, for example, nearly $4 billion was spent on these services, a figure five times greater than the actual cost of production. Pricing, redundancy, dual distribution and returned goods are aspects of the problem discussed. The cost of a drug promotion program is the major factor in overpricing and most of what is paid out in promotional expenses results in producer sovereignty. Also, drug prices are often inflated by 25 per cent to recover what has been spent on promotion. Irrational pricing is an added problem. Redundancy manifests itself in the excessive number of agents with similar therapeutic actions, as well as in the manufacture of the same product with marketing under different names, etc.

Another source of inefficiency in drug distribution is the result of making drugs available both on a direct basis and through wholesale suppliers. Finally, allowing purchasers to return merchandise for credit or replacement creates inefficiency because of the costs of handling and processing. There is a need here to study various aspects of the problem, including computer-managed inventories. Other factors influence the high cost of drug distribution as well and in order to have prices reflect more accurately the cost of production and distribution, there must either be a complete revamping of the free enterprise profit system or the development of new methods to work within the existing private enterprise system.

References, 18.

RUCKER, T. DONALD. *Inquiry 9 (3)*:43–50, September 1972.

1971

Pharmacy and the Poor

1 This is a report on the first two years of a project on pharmacy services for neighborhood health centers, funded by the Office of Economic Opportunity. Residents of poverty areas and the pharmacies available to them were surveyed in five urban locations and one rural location. Few differences were found between poor and nonpoor residents and between poverty area and nonpoverty area pharmacies in terms of size and number of prescriptions dispensed, age of pharmacist, prices charged for selected prescriptions and services requested from the pharmacist. The pharmacist was not viewed as a person to consult for advice on health matters. Pharmacy systems examined included health centers with on-site pharmacies staffed by more than one pharmacist using the team approach to health care, health centers with on-site pharmacies staffed by more than two pharmacists and having a high daily prescription volume, health centers which purchased pharmaceutical services from community pharmacies, and prepaid group medical practices with their own pharmacies. An on-site pharmacy does not always mean greater services for patients or prescribers, greater convenience for patients, an expanded role for the pharmacist, or an adverse economic impact on area pharmacies. An on-site pharmacy does mean low cost to the health center per prescription, greater opportunity for control, and greater educational and professional potential for the pharmacist. An off-site pharmacy means greater cost, more effort required for program controls, and a favorable economic impact on contractors.

References, 44.

AMERICAN PHARMACEUTICAL ASSOCIATION. Washington, D.C., The Association, 1971.

The Relative Stability of Drug Prices and Pharmacists' Fees

22

A comparative analysis of medical care service charges showed that the cost of drugs and prescriptions as well as pharmacist fees were the only two items among medical services that remained relatively stable during the period between 1963 and 1969. Since the Consumer Price Index only measures physicians' fees and optometrists' fees, the Kentucky Prescription Surveys were utilized and the figures generalized for the entire country as being indicative of an overall trend during that time period.

Wide variations in price increase were noted within medical care services, with the service charge for hospital rooms increasing more rapidly than any other service. In contrast to this, the cost of drugs and prescriptions remained almost stable, with only a 0.5 per cent increase that includes both prescription and over-the-counter drugs. Too, pharmacist fees rose only 10 per cent as noted in the Survey, while physicians' fees rose most rapidly at 35.8 per cent.

The rapid rise in the cost of medical care may be explained through an increase in the quality of care, an increase in the salaries of hospital workers, and in the rise of health-care programs as typified by Medicare. On the other hand, the stability of pharmacy products and services is explained by a slower rate of salary increase for pharmacy workers, increasing competition of drug sales in nonpharmacy stores, and close government scrutiny of the drug industry. However, whatever the causal factors may be, the notable fact is that the cost of drugs and prescriptions and pharmacists' fees were the only element of medical care services to remain stable in the period of 1963–1969.

References, 18. *Key words:* Reimbursement.

BILLUPS, NORMAN F.; and McGEE, L. RANDOLPH. *Journal of the American Pharmaceutical Association NS 11* (*1*):22–25, January 1971.

Health Insurance and Prescription Drugs

113

The ever increasing effectiveness of prescription drug products and the resulting confidence in the efficacy of drug treatment among physicians and patients help explain the rapidly growing use of prescription drugs. Various public and private health insurance plans covering prescription drugs are described. The major components of the drug industry are explained (manufacturers, wholesalers, retailers, pharmacists), and prescription drug prices for 1950–1968 are examined. Expenditures for prescription drugs have increased with rising consumer incomes and the availability of greater numbers of pharmaceuticals.

The fact that the percentage of total health care expenditures for prescription drugs has decreased in recent years may be explained by the great increase in hospital care expenditures, thus reducing the proportion available for other health services. In 1968, approximately 40 per cent of the United States civilian population had some form of outpatient prescription drug coverage, and $127 million in benefits were paid under major medical policies. Insurance plans are described in terms of eligibility, choice of prescriber and vendor, benefits, reimbursement and patient cost sharing. Most plans paid the insured directly, on the basis of the "reasonable retail price," but few companies kept cost and utilization data. Problems of controlling costs, drug quality and utilization are discussed.

References, 53. *Key words:* Patient cost sharing, reimbursement.

JONES, DONALD J.; and FOLLMAN, J.F. Washington, D.C., Health Insurance Association of America, 1971.

Basic Methods for Optimizing the Rational Prescribing of Psychoactive Drugs

190

The effective prescribing of psychoactive drugs (or of drug products in general) depends on (1) a national computer-assisted drug information network and data bank to record prescription orders and cope with third-party insurance claims, (2) systematic drug utilization review programs to evaluate prescription drug records for conformity to scientific standards for rational prescribing, dispensing and use (perhaps including cost considerations in addition to therapeutic considerations), and (3) a coordinated, systemic, objective information and education service ("a compendium system") for health care professionals.

Standards for rational prescribing should deal with factors such as (1) minimum and maximum drug quantities, appropriate dosages and strengths, refills, and adverse reactions, (2) criteria for no drug therapy or delayed drug therapy, (3) relationship of patient condition, age and sex to drug prescribing. With psychoactive drugs, the preparation of standards is difficult because guidelines for their efficacy are not yet available, standards for appropriate diagnosis must be developed and a concurrent review information system must be employed (while the patient is being examined) for feedback on therapeutic histories and standards. To counteract inappropriate prescribing and differences in prescribing habits, a compendium system, like drug utilization review, would be useful and should include a comprehensive reference work on all drug products marketed in the United States, selected information sources by therapeutic category or drug product, and an educational component (perhaps a committee to inform physicians about rational prescribing of specific products). These techniques could save more than $1 billion annually. However, certain marketing practices must be discontinued if unbiased and comprehensive information on drug therapy is to be provided.

References, 6.

RUCKER, T. DONALD. *Journal of Drug Issues 1* (3):326–332, Fall 1971.

Possible Impact of Government Drug Program on Community Pharmacies

196

A theoretical model is used to outline four general administrative requirements which might be associated with a federal program of prescription insurance coverage. The impact on community pharmacy operations is assessed as a result of each of the four requirements, which are: (1) to optimize patient care, (2) to minimize benefit and administrative outlays, (3) to ensure prudent fiscal management and (4) to ensure fiscal predictability or adherence to budget allocations. The theme recurring in each of the four analyses is that the administration of a drug benefit program is very complex and would require major improvements in the measurement and accounting of expenses associated with the dispensing functions of the pharmacy.

In order to achieve the first objective, the optimization of patient care, the pharmacist would have three roles: (1) to participate in review programs conducted by the drug insurance company, (2) to consult with patients concerning the proper use of medications, and (3) to interpret patient drug histories. The second objective, to minimize program outlays, would require that cost accounting procedures be improved in pharmacies in order to obtain an objective measurement of the economic value of the pharmacist, since reimbursement for services would be established by the third party insurer. A new system for submitting and processing drug insurance claims would need to be created before prescription benefits could be provided under a large government program. The third objective, prudent management, would require, due to the volume of claims anticipated, the use of a computer terminal to promptly transmit claim data directly to a central computer. The final objective, to ensure fiscal responsibility, would require that drug program expenditures be restricted, to the degree possible, to budget allocations. The issue of fiscal predictability may become less important if the drug insurance program is fulfilling the first three criteria.

References, 3. *Key words:* Drug utilization review.

RUCKER, T. DONALD. *Journal of the American Pharmaceutical Association NS11* (6):334–337, June 1971.

Prescription Drug Insurance for the Elderly under Medicare

234

The following five measures should precede or accompany prescription drug insurance under Medicare to help alleviate the particularly heavy burden of drug expenses borne by the elderly. These measures would promote appropriate prescribing, discourage excessive prescribing and upgrade the safety and efficacy of available drugs.

(1) The FDA should be given authority to restrict the marketing of new drugs to those judged by panels of experts to be as safe and more efficacious than any drug already available for the same indication. This system has held prescription drug entities in Norway to 1,200, while the United States has a confusing, largely duplicative, and often poorly tested melange of 5,000 prescription drugs and 21,000 "drug products."

(2) A government-sponsored drug compendium should provide expert panel discussions of drugs in therapeutic categories under generic names, as

an alternative to the manufacturer-oriented *Physicians' Desk Reference.* The discussion of digitalis from the National Academy of Sciences—National Research Council Drug Efficacy Study is appended as a model.

(3) Hospitals should have formularies and drug utilization review committees to cut down on adverse drug reactions and to control, through education and restraint, the excessive prescribing of antibiotics and other drugs. Computer-based prescription record systems, which can also help with inventory control and reordering, will be necessary.

(4) The federal government should provide more funds for training clinical pharmacologists, basic drug research and demonstration projects, and for the development of clinical pharmacology centers providing medical and continuing education on the clinical uses of drugs.

(5) Pharmacists should develop a new role as therapy advisors, to serve as liaison between patient and physician in drug therapy matters and to provide up-to-date drug information to prescribers. There have been several favorably received demonstrations of this innovation.

References, 8. *Key words:* Drug utilization review, formularies, other countries.

STOLLEY, PAUL, D.; and GODDARD, JAMES, L. *American Journal of Public Health 61* (3):574–581, March 1971.

1970

17 Problems Facing Pharmacists under Medicare and Medicaid

Dr. Apple outlines problems regarding payment for services provided under Medicare and Medicaid and offers possible solutions for these problems. The pharmacist's role in the task of drug use review is discussed at length.

This article is a reprint of a statement of the American Pharmaceutical Association to the Subcommittee on Medicare and Medicaid of the Senate Committee on Finance, June 16, 1970. Problems confronting the pharmacist under Medicare and Medicaid are classified into four areas: (1) inability to obtain prompt reimbursement from fiscal intermediaries, (2) inability to collect from institutional providers of health care who contracted for pharmaceutical services, e.g., nursing homes, (3) ethical and legal problems in the area of kickbacks to health care facilities, a practice deemed necessary in order to obtain contracts for pharmaceutical services and (4) abuses arising out of physician ownership of pharmaceutical facilities.

The problem of the time delay in receiving reimbursement is compounded by the fact that more than 50 per cent of the total claim amount represents reimbursement for the cost of the drug product, which was paid for in advance by the pharmacist. Due to "out-of-pocket" expenses, the pharmacist is often forced to borrow money to meet current operating expenses, a practice which adds to his financial burden since he is not compensated for the cost of borrowing. Pharmacists encounter additional severe difficulties when an across-the-board percentage reduction on the claims of Medicaid providers is imposed by the state. Such a reduction substantially reduces the pharmacist's compensation for his services, due to the fixed cost of the drug product.

Two solutions are advanced to solve problems in the area of reimbursement by health care providers: (1) certification by the provider that all suppliers' claims were paid before the provider would receive Medicare and Medicaid funds or (2) direct reimbursement to the supplier by the fiscal intermediary. This latter solution would, in addition, help to remedy the problem of kickback payments by the pharmacist to the health care provider. Since it is impossible to monitor the charges for the 12.5 million prescriptions dispensed annually to extended health care facilities, Dr. Apple proposes that the government require that compensation for pharmaceutical services be based on two components: (1) reimbursement for the cost of the drug and (2) a specified professional fee for the pharmacist's services. A plan employing these two principles devised by the Kansas Pharmaceutical Association and the Kansas Department of Social Welfare is described in detail. Finally, the problems connected with physician ownership of pharmaceutical services are discussed in connection with Senate bill 1575, which would prohibit federal financial participation in the cost of drugs under any program in which the medical practitioner has a financial interest in dispensing pharmaceuticals.

The American Pharmaceutical Association's reason for full support of the proposed legislation centers about abuses which occur in such situations and the undermining of the professionalism of pharmacists in situations where a physician controls the selection and dispensing of drugs. The Senate testimony concludes with comments on the pharmacist's role in drug utilization review; his contribution to the assurance of rational drug prescribing and dispensing practices and his contribution as the most knowledgeable source of information on program costs and administrative burdens in third-party programs.

References, 0. *Key words:* Drug utilization review.

APPLE, WILLIAM S. *Journal of the American Pharmaceutical Association NS10* (9):494–500, September 1970.

The New Handbook of Prescription Drugs: Official Names, Prices, and Sources for Patient and Doctor

36

This book discusses the characteristics of the drug industry; drug product testing and safety; relationships among the drug industry, physicians and medical schools and the consequent ethical problems; rational prescribing; generic versus brand name drugs and their relationship to unnecessary expenditures of Medicaid/Medicare funds; and the need for a national drug label law. Approximately 60 basic drugs, used to treat more than 90 per cent of adult outpatients, are reviewed. The bulk of the book is an alphabetical prescription drug list (brand name cross-referenced with generic name) offering commentary and the active ingredients and amounts in each dosage unit. Comparative prices are included for each manufacturer of a particular drug product. Appendices cover prescribing for children, the top 200 drugs in 1967 and the addresses of some distributors of generic drugs.

References, not counted; footnotes used.

BURACK, RICHARD. New York, Ballantine Books, 1970.

Controls over Medicaid Drug Program in Ohio Need Improvement

44

To evaluate the controls established to safeguard Ohio's Medicaid drug program from improper use, the General Accounting Office examined selected case records from the state department of public welfare, two county welfare departments, selected nursing homes and pharmacies. The state policy of paying pharmacies for drugs dispensed was studied for whether prices paid for selected drugs were reasonable and whether adequate records of drugs administered in nursing homes and dispensed by pharmacies were being kept. Information provided by the state to counties for caseworker determinations of drug usage was reviewed. Agencies were informed of the results of the study.

It was found that certain drugs were not reasonably priced because the state policy of paying pharmacies cost-plus-a-percentage-of-cost gave them an incentive for selling higher cost drug products. Controls for ensuring that prices billed to the state conformed to state regulations were inadequate. Nursing homes were not obtaining long-term maintenance drugs in economical quantities. It is recommended that federal assistance be provided to the states for revising their drug payment policies. Guidelines should be issued for drug utilization review, and their implementation should be monitored. Priority should be given to drug efficacy studies on those drug products identified by the HEW Task Force on Prescription Drugs as having the greatest potential for savings; results should be widely disseminated to physicians.

References, 0. *Key words:* Drug utilization review.

COMPTROLLER GENERAL OF THE UNITED STATES. Washington, D.C., Comptroller General, 1970.

Bibliography of Theses and Dissertations Relevant to Pharmacy Administration

126

This is an annotated bibliography of 400 masters theses and 350 Ph.D. dissertations, through December 1968, with author, title, degree, school, year, number of pages, and University Microfilm documentation and costs. Included are author and title indexes. Entries on pharmacy are presented in the following sections: pharmacy and pharmacists, pharmaceutical education, drugs, pharmaceutical industry, wholesaling, retail pharmacy operations, chain-store pharmacy, hospital pharmacy, history and law. Entries on related subjects are grouped in the following sections: health, administrative sciences, social sciences and humanities, the chemical industry.

See abstract 80, page 19.

KNAPP, DAVID A., Editor. Silver Spring, Maryland, American Association of Colleges of Pharmacy, 1970.

In 1968 . . . Insurance Paid an Estimated $125 Million for Medications

10

A recent Health Insurance Institute estimate put benefits for drugs and medications under major medical insurance policies at $125 million in 1968. The final figure for 1967 was $109 million. Over 62 million Americans have major medical insurance, and nearly 59 million under age 65 are covered for prescribed drugs and special nursing care. Nursing care expenses increased $10 million to $78 million from 1966 to 1967. There was also a significant increase in hospital, medical and surgical expenses, which represents the bulk of major medical payments. The highest item—hospital care—rose $89 million in 1967 to $595 million; major medical payments increased $53 million to $355 million; and surgical expenses, $41 million to $278 million. Other benefits went from $22 million in 1966 to $26 million in 1967. Overall, American families received over $1.4 billion in payments in 1967 and the estimate for 1968 is $1.62 billion. Major medical policies usually pay 75 per cent or 80 per cent of bills (up to a maximum) after a deductible amount of $50 to $500.

References, 0.

ANONYMOUS. *American Professional Pharmacist* 35 (3):40–41, March 1969.

Under Tax Supported Programs. Cost of Providing Pharmaceuticals

19

The contention that it is cheaper to dispense prescribed drugs through hospital pharmacies is supported by a comparative cost analysis but challenged in terms of service standards. Cost data for providing "forty representative drugs" were gathered from two large government hospitals, one county and one federal, and from a county welfare vendor program. The mean dispensing cost for pharmacy outpatient operations, computed by dividing direct and indirect costs by number of prescription orders, came to $.63 for the county hospital (1965) and $.94 for the federal one (1966), not including significant mailing costs for the latter. Drug costs were $3.36 and $2.57 for sole-source products and $1.07 and $1.17 for drugs available from multiple sources. Dispensing and drug costs for the vendor pharmacies were based on the county's public assistance pricing schedule, with dispensing cost varying with medication cost. The dispensing cost was $2.36 with a drug cost of $2.99 for sole-source drugs and $1.59 with $1.49 for multiple-source ones. When the data were adjusted for quantity dispensed and prescription mix, the county hospital drug costs dropped to $2.28 and $.67 for the two categories and the federal costs to $1.67 and $.56.

The reasons for lower hospital dispensing costs may include the greater use of nonprofessionals, prepackaged products, a smaller selection and a lack of the need to get renewal authorizations, provide information on nonprescribed drugs, or rush so much at peak hours. These factors lower the level of service along with the costs. The hospital's lower drug costs result from special hospital and government discounts plus quantity purchasing and the use of competitive bids. It may be that highly trained hospital pharmacists are being diverted from the inpatient services they provide most effectively. A hospital with outpatient dispensing must have a high standard of inpatient service while providing a level of outpatient service characterized by such criteria as pharmacist explanation of directions to patients, fulfillment of legal requirements, accurate patient records, minimum waiting periods for prescriptions, direct or indirect supply of all medicinal adjuncts, delivery on request, provision for emergency service, health information availability and convenient location. Essentials like the first two form the basic unit for reimbursement; others could be optional and justify additional charges. Costs to be summed should include social costs, like patient time. Low dispensing costs are not equivalent to proper service.

References, 13. *Key words:* Reimbursement.

BACHYNSKY, JOHN A.; and HAMMEL, ROBERT W. *Journal of the American Pharmaceutical Association NS 9 (6)*:269–272, June 1969.

A Publicly Funded Pharmacy Program under Medicaid in New York City

120

The New York City Medicaid Pharmacy Program is the largest in the country. It now includes 2,330 pharmacies, representing 71 per cent of the city's total. From 1934 to 1966, public assistance pharmacy services were provided by the City Welfare Department. Its panel of physicians was encouraged to prescribe generic drugs and pharmacists needed special authorization for any drug above $2.25. Reimbursement was based on drug cost plus a sliding scale mark-up. Few complaints about the stringent controls were received, perhaps because relatively little money was involved. Transition to the Medicaid pharmacy program was complex because of growth, shared responsibilities with the Department of Health, and the fact that Medicaid enrollees can select their own providers. Only pharmacy invoices over $20 now require prior approval. An Advisory Committee on Quality Pharmacy sets reimbursement standards and policies.

Following heated disputes among the State and City Health Departments and affected professionals, generic substitution is now possible only when a prescriber explicitly authorizes it. The Medicaid formulary lists 1200 drugs with computer codes. The percentages of participating pharmacies, which tend to remain in the program, ranged in 1967–68 from 52.4 in Manhattan to 81.5 in the Bronx, with a city-wide average of 10 pharmacies per 10,000 Medicaid enrollees. Prescribers use a special Prescription Order and Invoice form. Reimbursement is based on cost plus $66\frac{2}{3}$ per cent (50 per cent since June 1969).

There are limits on the length of supply and the number of refills allowed. The pharmacist submits an invoice copy to the Department of Social Services and is reimbursed twice monthly after a sample audit. Payment has just risen from 95 per cent to 100 per cent of face value. Payments to pharmacies in 1968 were almost $18 million, which represented 12 per cent of all payments to private health care practitioners and an average of $7,710 per pharmacy. Over 4 million invoices were processed at an average cost, based on a one-day sample, of $3.59 per prescription. The Health Department is responsible for monitoring and enforcement, and the Department of Social Services and the

State Board of Pharmacy participate in the watchdog system. Prescription examination and on-site spot checks have uncovered some irregularities, and patient complaints even more, but the percentage is relatively small. There have been major problems with late, and sometimes poorly documented, payments, but these have been mostly overcome. The Medicaid Administration favors the development of a formulary system to promote generic substitution. It would also prefer going from a mark-up to a professional fee system, which pharmacists seem to like but which is still subject to debate.

References, 13. *Key words:* Formularies, reimbursement, substitution.

KAVALER, FLORENCE; BELLIN, LOWELL E.; GREEN, ALEX; GORELIK, ELIHU A.; and ALEXANDER, RAYMOND S. *Medical Care* 7 (5):361–371, September–October 1969.

The Pharmaceutical Revolution: Its Impact on Science and Society

139

Scientific and technological advances resulting in the "pharmaceutical revolution" include (1) increased knowledge of disease processes, (2) greater knowledge of drug action (positive and negative), and (3) expanded facilities and resources for drug screening, production and marketing in private, government and academic sectors. These developments have led to personal expectations of improved medical care, health and life span, as well as economic expectations of less lost work time due to illness. In large measure, these have been fulfilled.

There are problems, however, such as serious side effects of potent new drugs, drug interactions, overtreatment, unethical behavior in clinical investigations and the moral dilemma involving the goals of society versus the good of the individual. Action from organizations such as the FDA, the National Academy of Sciences, state legislatures and other federal and international regulatory agencies has been required to protect patients and to involve them in medical decision making. National and international networks for data on drug efficacy and toxicity are needed, along with computer-based correlations of patient characteristics and drug response, so that drug treatment can be predictable and individualized. Drug utilization review and standards of drug quality and effectiveness ("physiological availability") are also required; new biological testing procedures can be utilized.

References, 19. *Key words:* Drug utilization review.

LASAGNA, LOUIS. *Science 166 (3910)*:1227–1233, December 5, 1969.

The Economic Impact of Third Party Payment for Drugs

173

Blue Cross introduced drug prepayment as part of an integrated collection of health benefits in order to meet public demands for in-depth health care protection for all health services. Blue Cross contracts with participating pharmacies to pay acquisition costs plus reasonable dispensing fees. A majority of the pharmacies in a given area must participate in order for the plan to be successful. Costs are constantly reviewed. Copayments range from 25¢ to $2.00. Coverage of some drug products, such as oral contraceptives, is optional. No position has been taken (1969) on requiring generic drugs. It is expected that the use of prepayment drug plans will increase the time spent by pharmacists on professional duties. Until prepayment covers one-fifth to one-third of the market, the economic impact will not be widely felt. This point is expected to be reached in several years.

References, 0. *Key words:* Patient cost sharing.

PEARCE, H.G. *Medical Marketing and Media* 4 (*11*):25–26, 28–29, November 1969.

Approaches to Drug Insurance Design

239 This background paper includes a study of some of the chief elements involved in designing a drug insurance program. It also presents various alternatives for consideration when developing such a program. The volume includes chapters on the making of the blueprint; scope of benefit; program financing; reimbursement; methods of patient cost sharing; program administration; classification and coding; utilization review; and program estimates. It is liberally referenced and contains 15 tables of data.

References, not counted; footnotes used. *Key words:* Drug utilization review, formularies, patient cost sharing, reimbursement.

TASK FORCE ON PRESCRIPTION DRUGS. Background Papers. Office of the Secretary. United States Department of Health, Education and Welfare. Washington, D.C., United States Government Printing Office, 1969.

Final Report

244 The Task Force was established in May 1967 to undertake a comprehensive study of the problems of including the costs of prescription drugs under the Medicare program. The Task Force Master Drug List contained the 409 most frequently prescribed drugs dispensed to the elderly in 1966, accounting for 88 per cent of all prescriptions dispensed by community pharmacies for the elderly, and 88 per cent of the pharmacies' retail prescription drug costs. More than 90 per cent of the products were dispensed under brand names; 86 of these had cheaper chemical equivalents available.

The report recommends legislation requiring all dispensed prescription drugs to be labeled with identity, strength and quantity of product. It supports the idea of increased information for consumers on local prescription prices, discusses clinical and biological equivalency and recommends uniform standards of quality and efficacy for drugs in any federally-supported program. The report concludes that the use of low-cost chemical equivalents can yield important savings in certain therapeutic categories; this use should be encouraged wherever consistent with high quality medical care.

The Task Force found the average prescription prices in welfare programs to be approximately 10 per cent lower in formulary states and where required in federal programs (military, Veterans Administration and Public Health Service hospitals, in-hospital care under Medicare). In general, American physicians find a formulary acceptable and practical if designed and maintained by clinical and scientific colleagues, if quality is considered as being as important as price, and if provisions are made for prescribing unlisted drug products. Drug costs can also be controlled by limiting the maximum quantities dispensed and the number of permitted refills. The exclusion of certain combination products, duplicative drugs and noncritical products (for example, antacids) from federal reimbursement programs contributes significantly to rational prescribing and cost savings. The report recommends the establishment of reasonable cost and charge ranges for drugs provided under federal programs, drug utilization review and copayment.

References, not counted; footnotes used. *Key words:* Formularies, patient cost sharing, reimbursement, substitution.

TASK FORCE ON PRESCRIPTION DRUGS. Office of the Secretary. United States Department of Health, Education, and Welfare. Washington, D.C., United States Government Printing Office, 1969.

1968

The Relationship of Drug Costs to Medical Care

28

Drug prices rose in the period 1965–67, but not as fast as other health care items. Twelve per cent (1967) of the country's public and private health expenditures goes for drug products. Increasing drug consumption can be related to the use of drug products as the basic means of treatment and to the longer lifespans of people with chronic conditions that require drug treatment.

The Consumer Price Index (CPI) for prescription drugs shows a decline for 1957–67, yet total and per capita consumer drug expenditures are rising. This indicates increases in the number of prescriptions per person and in the average cost of a prescription. Price trends for 1957–67 (base year 1965) for the 200 most frequently prescribed drugs were studied (representing two-thirds of the prescription dollar market), using wholesale prices from the *Drug Topics Red Book.* For the 1965 drug list, 57 of the 200 drugs showed price increases since 1957; 27 drugs showed price decreases. This does not support the decline in the CPI for prescription drugs. However, of the 200 most frequently prescribed drugs studied, 53 per cent were introduced after 1957; of the drugs in the CPI, only 14 per cent were introduced after 1957. Thus, the CPI is not representative of the drug market. The prices of 31 drugs added to the list of the 200 most frequently prescribed drugs between 1963 and 1965 were compared with the prices of the 31 drugs dropped from the list. The newer drugs were more costly. Also, replacement drugs by therapeutic category are generally more expensive. With insurance benefits for drug expenses growing, pharmacists should actively support cost-benefit analysis of drug problems. This technique considers social and economic as well as medical factors and is especially valuable with problems such as national immunization programs.

References, 0.

BREWSTER, AGNES W.; and HORTON, JUANITA P. *American Journal of Hospital Pharmacy* 25 (4):176–179, April 1968.

The Drug Makers and the Drug Distributors

241 As part of the major HEW study on the problems involved in including prescription drug costs under Medicare, the production and distribution of drugs were examined. Issues discussed include the "big business" nature of drug manufacturers, changes in competitive practices in the 1960's, patents and trademarks, research and development activities, the growth of federally-financed health care programs, quality control and federal regulation, marketing and pricing practices, and profitability and risk in the drug industry. The roles of drug wholesalers and different types of pharmacies are discussed along with pharmacy regulation. The drug industry is reported to spend: (1) a higher proportion of corporate funds on research than any other industry; and (2) approximately one-fourth of each sales dollar on marketing and advertising. This report contains 17 tables and 16 figures.

References, 131.

TASK FORCE ON PRESCRIPTION DRUGS. Background Papers. Office of the Secretary. United States Department of Health, Education, and Welfare. Washington, D.C., United States Government Printing Office. 1968.

The Drug Prescribers

242 The HEW Task Force on Prescription Drugs investigated: (1) the prescribing patterns of physicians, their training and their information sources on drugs; (2) questions of drug quality (chemical, biological and clinical equivalence, drug standards and quality control); and (3) the use of formularies or drug lists. The various therapeutic judgments that must be made by drug prescribers are described, along with the teaching of pharmacology as a clinical science in several United States medical schools.

The ways in which physicians receive information are examined; for example, medical journals, drug compendia, textbooks, industry advertising, detail men and drug samples. In one study, 57 per cent of 141 physicians indicated that the initial source of information about a new drug was the detail man. In another study, 85 per cent of the physicians reported great confidence in the information provided by detail men.

Various aspects of the drug equivalency controversy are presented. Brand-name manufacturers claim to have quality control standards higher than those of low-cost generic drug manufacturers. The *United States Pharmacopeia* and *National Formulary* are described and assessed and found adequate for their purposes. The responsibilities of the FDA and the Division of Biologic Standards are described. The development of various formularies and drug lists are described.

References, 92. *Key words:* Substitution.

TASK FORCE ON PRESCRIPTION DRUGS. Background Papers. Office of the Secretary. United States Department of Health, Education, and Welfare. Washington, D.C., United States Government Printing Office, 1968.

The Drug Users

243 The HEW Task Force on Prescription Drugs was established in 1967 to undertake a comprehensive study of the problems of including the cost of prescription drugs under Medicare. This volume in the background papers series deals with the health needs of the elderly, including data and discussions related to their financial resources, expenditure patterns, and use of prescribed drugs.

Demographic information on the elderly population (those 65 or older) is presented, including breakdowns by age, sex and level of education. Additional information is provided about financial assets, current income and income sources, and the number and distribution of the elderly poor.

The health needs of this segment of the population are discussed. The discussion includes a presentation of data by type of service, the amount and distribution of expenditures for prescribed drugs, and the methods of paying for health care services including insurance, tax relief and out-of-pocket cost.

Extensive data are presented on patterns of drug use. The Task Force created a master prescription drug list consisting of the 409 products most frequently used by the elderly. Use and cost data are provided on each of the products on the master drug list. The report concludes with a discussion of the importance of maintenance drug therapy to the elderly, and the issue of generic prescribing.

References, not counted; footnotes used. *Key words:* Drug utilization review.

TASK FORCE ON PRESCRIPTION DRUGS. Background papers. Office of the Secretary. United States Department of Health, Education and Welfare. Washington, D.C., United States Government Printing Office, 1968.

1967

Prepaid Drug Plans Sponsored by Pharmacists

64

The article explores the development in the late 1950's and 1960's of prepaid drug plans sponsored by pharmacists in Canada and the United States, and comments on the feasibility and future of first-dollar prescription drug coverage. In pharmacy-sponsored plans, the pharmacists act both as the providers of services and as the organizers and controllers of the plan. The plans described, in great detail, are: (1) Prescription Services, Inc. (Canada), (2) Pharmacare, Ltd., a program planned (1966) by the American Pharmaceutical Association, (3) Prescription Services, Inc. (California) and (4) California Pharmaceutical Services. Some short-lived plans sponsored by Blue Cross organizations are discussed briefly.

For all plans, the discussion emphasizes the mode of financing, the groups eligible for coverage, the extent of benefit coverage and the plan's success. The position of the Federal Trade Commission, that pharmacy-sponsored prepaid drug plans could be in violation of the Sherman Antitrust Act, is discussed and evaluated. The reasons for the promotion by pharmacists of prepaid drug plans in the mid 1960's are outlined. The existence of Medicare and Medicaid is seen as a boost to the provision of prepaid plans for all groups of persons.

Fletcher concludes that future prepaid plans should be underwritten by private insurance companies. Principles to consider in the development of a prepaid drug program include: (1) the need to enlist the support of pharmacists and pharmaceutical associations, (2) the need to limit coverage to groups of substantial size, (3) the need to include first-dollar drug coverage as part of existing coverage, via a rider policy, (4) the need to limit the size of the prescription for which benefits would be payable, (5) the need to have a stated deductible and (6) the need to have a maximum amount of reimbursement available over a particular time period.

References, 18. *Key words:* Other countries, patient cost sharing.

FLETCHER, LINDA P. *Journal of Risk and Insurance* 34 (*1*):81–94, March 1967.

1966

Study of Drug Purchase Problems and Policies

43

This review provides information on legislation and related research reports plus data on prescriptions for 1952–1963. It discusses the volume and cost of drugs; standard sources of drug information and evaluation; patents, drug names and trademarks; generic prescribing and formularies in the reduction of drug costs; alternative methods of drug distribution; British drug programs; and managing drugs in public assistance programs.

References, 52. *Key words:* Formularies, other countries, patents and prices.

CLAPP, RAYMOND F. Welfare Research Report 2. United States Department of Health, Education and Welfare. Washington, D.C., United States Government Printing Office, March 1966.

1964

Patterns of Drug Use by Type in a Prepaid Medical Plan

26

The cost and utilization experience under a prepaid drug benefit is described and analyzed in terms of the therapeutic purpose of the medications prescribed. The program studied was that of the Group Health Association (GHA), Washington, D.C., for the benefit year 1960–61. The program applied to persons in the GHA premium plan (26,954) who incurred more than $25 in prescription drug expenses in the twelve-month period. Most of the members of GHA were employed persons and their dependents, so there is relatively less data available on drugs commonly used by older persons. A total of 8,919 individual prescriptions of a sample population of 515 claimants who filed valid claims were analyzed and classified into fourteen specific therapeutic categories, one category combining several relatively uncommon types, and an unclassified group.

The distributional analysis showed that the anti-infective category of drugs was the most frequently prescribed (13.3 per cent), while more than 10 per cent of prescriptions were for psychotropic (10.6 per cent) and cardiovascular (10.4 per cent) drugs. Although GHA physicians were not at the time urged to prescribe by generic name, 12.2 per cent of all prescriptions were written by generic name. The highest percentage of refills was for psychotropic drugs. The average refill ratio for all drug classes was 37.5 per cent, compared with 48.2 per cent nation-wide, as determined by *American Druggist* surveys. Several reasons which could account for the variance are given.

The data are also analyzed to show the per cent distribution of claimants according to the number of prescriptions, by therapeutic type, received. The expenditures for drugs are detailed by therapeutic class. The average prescription price for all drugs of $4.21 was higher than the national average as determined in several surveys (e.g., *American Druggist,* average price of $3.22, 1961). Prescriptions were additionally analyzed for percentage of therapeutic class contained in dollar price intervals and in terms of sex and age categories. Claimants under 19 had proportionally the greatest number of prescriptions under $5. The age-specific patterns found were generally indicative of the type of illness affecting each age group.

References, 7. *Key words:* Patient cost sharing, substitution.

BREWSTER, AGNES W.; ALLEN, SCOTT I.; and HOLEN, ARLENE. *Public Health Reports* 79 (5):403–409, May 1964.

1963
Experience with a Prepaid Drug Benefit

27

The first year's experience (during 1960–61) with the prepaid drug program of Group Health Association, Inc. (GHA), Washington, D.C., a prepayment group practice plan, was examined by the Division of Community Health Services of HEW. The program applies to persons in the GHA premium plan who incurred more than $25 in prescription drug expenses in a twelve-month period. Eighty per cent of the amount over the $25 deductible is reimbursable. The drug benefit applied to 27,274 persons. Two different aspects of the use of prescribed drugs are discussed: the actuarial aspects of the program, and the pharmaceutical aspects of drugs prescribed and average expenditures for drugs prescribed.

Some specific actuarial aspects determined were: (1) 4.5 per cent of the 27,274 eligible subscribers reported they had incurred charges of $25 or more; thus, there were 1,184 claimants, (2) the claimant rate rose by age group: 5.6 per cent of children under age 5 and 16.5 per cent of persons aged 65 and over were claimants, (3) there was almost no difference in claimant rates between subscribers (major members) and adult dependents (spouses), (4) the average number of prescriptions, including refills, was 16.7 per claimant; the rate rose with advancing age, and (5) overall reimbursement amounted to 51 per cent of the total expenditure for prescribed drugs by claimants.

The second part of the study analyzed the pharmaceutical aspects and expenditures for those drugs prescribed for the claimants. Forty-five percent of the 19,718 prescriptions allowed were analyzed. Some specific findings were: (1) the anti-infective category of drugs was the most prescribed (14 per cent) of the 14 drug categories. The pattern of drug use varied with the age group and reflected the type of illness common to each group, (2) only 15 per cent of the sample prescriptions were written for generic drugs, and (3) long-term therapy, as measured by the ratio of refills to total prescriptions, was most prevalent (54 per cent) for the psychotropic drug group. Five or more prescriptions per year were used by nearly 48 per cent of patients using cardiovascular and diuretic types of drugs.

References, 2. *Key words:* Patient cost sharing.

BREWSTER, AGNES W.; ALLEN, SCOTT I.; and KRAMER, LUCY M. *Journal of Health and Human Behavior* 4 (1):14–22, Spring 1963.

1961

Health Insurance for the Cost of Drugs

66

Studies show increases in the use and cost of drugs, in the proportion of the population having insurance protection, and in the coverage of prescription drugs (both in and out of hospital) by voluntary health insurance plans. Drug benefits range from 4–9 per cent of total benefits, depending on age, sex, economic level, amount of insurance deductible, and maturity of group insurance plan.

Data are presented for a large group plan for 1957–1959. As the plan matured and coverage was better understood, drug benefits rose from 7.45 per cent of total medical benefits to 8.98 per cent. Drug expenditures for salaried employees under the plan (10.59 per cent in 1959) exceeded those for hourly employees (7.48 per cent in 1959). Variables in voluntary health insurance plans include restrictions on choice of drug, choice of pharmacy, fees and eligibility. Some plans operate with labor union "nonprofit" pharmacies, where members can purchase drugs at 30 per cent savings. Other plans cover drugs on a deductible basis.

Prepaid drug coverage is considered an inefficient use of health insurance money and unacceptable to the public unless combined with total health care coverage. A prepaid prescription plan in Ontario, Canada, begun by pharmacists in 1958, has not been successful. The California Pharmaceutical Association plan, begun in 1959, has not yet been evaluated [article written in 1961]. Controls on utilization must be provided to avoid treatment that is unnecessary or more costly than required. Various types of control, such as formularies or centralized purchasing and distribution, have been instituted by public health agencies in the United States and other countries. Cooperation is required between the insurers, insured, physicians and pharmacists.

References, 11. *Key words:* Other countries, patient cost sharing.

FOLLMANN, J.F., JR. *American Journal of Public Health 51* (5):659–664, May 1961.

III

Experiences in Other Countries

Included are reports of drug-related cost control efforts in other countries. Key words: Other countries.

1977

Report from Canada

18

Canada's provincial governments are responsible for the health care programs developed in response to the needs of the different provinces. Most have pharmaceutical benefit programs for persons aged 65 and over. Several factors influenced the development of these programs. The federal government loosened patent protection, stimulating the number of competitive brands available, and implemented a drug quality assessment program. Provincial governments passed legislation allowing product selection by pharmacists (usually from a formulary), assumed control of municipal public assistance drug programs, and instituted a maximum fee for service plan. Pharmacists, through their professional associations, negotiated fees and services, and pharmacy licensing bodies monitored the program for the provincial government, acting in cases of fraud or unprofessional conduct. The federal government involvement is limited to drug quality. Private drug programs are growing slowly.

Formularies, where used, restrict benefits to those therapeutically acceptable drugs, set reimbursement rates and may list interchangeable products. Some provinces require a 20 per cent copayment; others require payment of a disbursing fee (approximately $2.00). The approaches of six provinces are discussed. Two provincial programs cover all residents; others cover elderly persons, welfare recipients, or low-income wage earners. In Manitoba, claim forms are usually completed by pharmacists at patient request, and patients submit the forms twice a year to receive payment. Claims processing costs are thus kept low. In Quebec, an extra charge is made for services provided between midnight and 7 a.m. Various methods of controlling drug ingredient costs have been tried, including formularies, committee rulings, price agreements with manufacturers and wholesalers, and product selection legislation.

References, 0. *Key words:* Formularies, patents and prices, patient cost sharing, reimbursement, substitution.

BACHYNSKY, J.A. *In* Wertheimer, Albert I., Editor. *Proceedings of the International Conference on Drug and Pharmaceutical Services Reimbursement.* Public Health Service. Health Resources Administration. National Center for Health Services Research. DHEW Publication No. (HRA) 77-3186. Springfield, Virginia, National Technical Information Service, June 1977. Pages 73–83.

Report from West Germany

97

Ninety-two per cent of the West German population belongs to statutory "sick funds," to which both employee and employer contribute. Pharmacies dispense drugs to insured persons for a 20 per cent charge (maximum charge approximately $1.07); pensioners, unemployed persons and hardship cases are exempt from this copayment. Publicly insured drug sales account for 60 per cent of total drug sales. Drug expenses amount to 15 per cent of the total cost of statutory health insurance plans. The statutory sick funds (about 1500 self-governing plans) negotiate fee structures with the medical profession. The sick funds and representative doctors support a federal committee on guidelines for drug prescriptions and prices. (Note: Costs have been converted from German Marks to United States dollars, based on the following exchange rate: 1 Mark equals $.43).

Prescribing is reviewed for quantity and quality. Maximum prices and price margins for drugs are fixed by government departments of economics and health, and recognize the interests of consumers as well as pharmacies. Prices are based on manufacturing costs, wholesale prices and additional charges made by pharmacies to realize gross earnings in the range of 25.9 per cent to 42.6 per cent. By law, pharmacists must grant sick funds a 5 per cent discount. There are legal requirements for persons who wish to establish pharmacies to insure that a balanced supply of drugs can be dispensed to all segments of the population by licensed and reliable persons. Pharmacies hold a monopoly on drug distribution and obtain their drugs from about 30 wholesalers. In general, pharmacies are supplied 3 times a day and must maintain a stock adequate to supply the population with drugs for 8 days. Items such as mineral waters, therapeutic sea salts, muds for mud baths, dressings and antiseptics are exempt from monopoly by law and can be dispensed by other establishments. The hospital system and special programs for the chronically ill are described.

References, 0. *Key words:* Drug utilization review, patient cost sharing, reimbursement.

HELMER, IRMELA. *In* Wertheimer, Albert I., Editor. *Proceedings of the International Conference on Drug and Pharmaceutical Services Reimbursement.* Public Health Service. Health Resources Administration. National Center for Health Services Research. DHEW Publication No. (HRA) 77-3186. Springfield, Virginia, National Technical Information Service, June 1977. Pages 29–36.

Report from Norway

110

The entire population of Norway is covered by compulsory health insurance programs administered by the 19 provinces and 444 local governments. Hospital treatment is free; medical care is available on a limited cost sharing basis. Drugs for long-term and chronic diseases, plus drugs used in hospitals, account for 60 per cent of total prescriptions. The establishment and geographic distribution of pharmacies, qualifications and licensing of pharmacy personnel, hours of service and restricted distribution of an adequate supply of drugs are controlled by law. Pharmacies in unfavorable (rural) locations are supported by tax incentives. Government guaranteed loans are available to qualified proprietor applicants. Drug wholesaling is controlled by government monopoly. Sales of pharmaceuticals are restricted to pharmacies, except where sparse population requires the dispensing of nonprescription medicines by other outlets.

Prescription drugs are dispensed in the manufacturers' original packages. Pharmacists have a 5-year university education, prescriptionists a $2\frac{1}{2}$ year education and technical assistants a special training program; prescriptionists may dispense medicines but may not own or manage a pharmacy. Government standards of therapeutic effectiveness and safety must be met before a medicine is registered for distribution. Registration is denied for duplicate products and for products lacking therapeutic or economic justification. These restrictions (allowing about 1200 products in 1850 dosage forms) permit physicians to work with a manageable number of drugs, and pharmacists to keep the necessary drugs in stock easily. They also lower total health care costs.

Drug tests, manufacturing practices (satisfactory storage and handling) and pharmacy premises and equipment are also government controlled, with periodic inspection of pharmacies and pharmaceutical industries. Drug advertising is limited to objective information and is prohibited on radio, television and in public places. In an effort to increase patient compliance with prescription requirements, pharmacists offer both verbal and written medical instructions. Retail drug prices are negotiated with manufacturers and reviewed periodically. Pharmacy dispensing fees are also fixed; this determines the average allowable annual income for pharmacy proprietors. The bookkeeping practices of pharmacies are also regulated.

References, 0. *Key words:* Reimbursement.

JØDAL, BJØRN. *In* Wertheimer, Albert I., Editor. *Proceedings of the International Conference on Drug and Pharmaceutical Services Reimbursement.* Public Health Service. Health Resources Administration. National Center for Health Services Research. DHEW Publication No. (HRA) 77-3186. Springfield, Virginia, National Technical Information Service, June 1977. Pages 105–120.

Drug Use in Australia and the United States as Reflections of Legislation and Social Attitudes

133

A comparison of drug use in the United States and Australia reveals similarities in drug marketing requirements, although the United States has stricter controls over prescription drugs and Australia has stricter controls over nonprescription drugs. The largest drug manufacturer in Australia is government-subsidized; the United States government does not market drugs. Australia's national Pharmaceutical Benefits Scheme (PBS), established in 1952, covers drugs for hospital patients (either in- or out-), and for veterans and pensioners free of charge; other nonhospital patients pay an A$2 copayment per prescription. The United States does not yet have a national drug benefits program.

The Australian PBS controls drug quality and use; a *Pharmaceutical Benefits* book, sent to physicians three times a year, lists accepted drugs, drug restrictions, maximum quantities and refills, approved prices and proper matching of drug and diagnosis. Computer-assisted review of physician prescribing at the national level may result in actions ranging from a letter of warning to the revocation of authority to prescribe under the PBS. Drug use review in the

United States under Professional Standards Review Organization programs is initiated at the local level.

The social approach to drug benefits differs. Whereas United States drug benefit programs have focused on the poor, aged, veterans and other special groups because of the large number of potential claims under a national scheme, the relatively small population of Australia has allowed that country to extend benefits to the entire population.

References, 5. *Key words:* Drug utilization review.

KNAPP, DAVID A.; KNAPP, DEANNE E.; and BROOKS, GEOFFREY E. *Drug Intelligence and Clinical Pharmacy 11* (5):298–303, May 1977.

Report from Sweden

149 National Health Insurance was established in Sweden in 1955 and covers hospital, medical, dental and maternity care, including pharmaceutical preparations, plus pensions and some special allowances. Coverage is provided for all Swedish citizens and for non-Swedish citizens who work and live in Sweden. Twenty-six regional offices administer the insurance system. All persons earning taxable income contribute to the health insurance fund. Patients treated by government doctors pay $3.60 per office visit or $6.00 per home visit. The telephone consultation charge is $2.40. These fees include x-rays and laboratory tests and the first visit, if referred to another doctor. There are no fees for inpatient hospital care. There is a system for the reimbursement of private physicians. (Note: Costs have been converted from Swedish Crowns to United States dollars, based on the following exchange rate: 1 Crown equals $0.24).

Drugs prescribed by doctors or dentists are dispensed by pharmacists free for patients with long-term or serious illnesses (the government decides which diseases and drugs qualify), or at a reduced price for other drugs, with a maximum outlay of $4.80 for all prescribed and registered drugs purchased at any one time. A list of drugs provided free of charge is included with this paper; commonly prescribed drugs in 29 disease categories are covered. During 1975, the cost of these drug benefits was 78.2 per cent of the total value of all filled prescriptions, and amounted to approximately $291 million. Of this, 17.4 per cent was for prescribed drugs dispensed free of charge and 82.6 per cent for drugs at reduced prices.

References, 0. *Key words:* Formularies, patient cost sharing.

LÖNNGREN, RUNE. *In* Wertheimer, Albert I., Editor. *Proceedings of the International Conference on Drug and Pharmaceutical Services Reimbursement.* Public Health Service. Health Resources Administration. National Center for Health Services Research. DHEW Publication No. (HRA) 77-3186. Springfield, Virginia, National Technical Information Service, June 1977. Pages 61–71.

Report from Australia

212 Medicine and pharmacy in Australia are controlled by the six states and two federal territories. All citizens have medical/hospital insurance through the government Medibank scheme or nonprofit insurance companies. The organization of the health care system is described. The federal health department is responsible for drug standards and testing and for pharmaceutical benefits. About 80 per cent of all prescription drugs are supplied to consumers through retail pharmacies and about 20 per cent through hospitals. Pharmacies purchase most pharmaceuticals from wholesalers who operate on a 15 per cent margin. Between 10–20 per cent are purchased directly from manufacturers, usually at a significant discount. About 90 per cent of dispensed prescriptions are covered by the government's Pharmaceutical Benefits Scheme, but allowable items account for less than half of the available drugs.

Pensioners receive prescription drugs free; others pay $2.00 per supply of a prescription. It is believed that the higher the patient contribution, the greater the deterrent effect on overutilization by patients and doctors; copayments have risen from $.50 in March 1960 to $2.00 in March 1976. The average value of a National Health prescription is $3.60; thus, pharmacists are reimbursed an average of $1.60 per prescription.

Ninety-five per cent of the benefit items dispensed are ready prepared; 5 per cent are mixed by the pharmacist to the doctor's specifications. Benefit pharmaceuticals must meet standards of quality, safety and efficacy, and be available at a satisfactory price. They may be available for unrestricted use or be restricted by specific diseases, users, purposes or quantities. Benefit drugs are reviewed periodically. The Pharmaceutical Benefits Advisory Committee (six doctors, two pharmacists, one pharmacologist) advises the federal health department on drug matters. Pharmacists submit prescription claims for reimbursement monthly. Pricing and processing (including quality control and doctor identification checks) are done by computer, and payment is made within two and a half weeks. Computer processing also allows analysis of prescribing and manufacturing practices and benefits. The health department and pharmaceutical manufacturers negotiate on prices for benefit items.

Retail drug prices are based on wholesale prices, a $33\frac{1}{3}$ per cent markup, a professional fee of $.84 and miscellaneous charges (for example, container allowance, dangerous drug fee). Health department pharmacists (armed with computer printouts of prescribing records) regularly visit doctors to advise against excessive prescribing and to answer questions; this program tries to counteract the promotional activities of drug manufacturers. Pharmacies are also visited.

References, 0. *Key words:* Drug utilization review, patient cost sharing, reimbursement.

SHIELDS, ARTHUR. *In* Wertheimer, Albert I., Editor. *Proceedings of the International Conference on Drug and Pharmaceutical Services Reimbursement.* Public Health Service. Health Resources Administration. National Center for Health Services Research. DHEW Publication No. (HRA) 77-3186. Springfield, Virginia, National Technical Information Service, June 1977. Pages 37–59.

Proceedings of the International Conference on Drug and Pharmaceutical Services Reimbursement

254

This conference was held in Washington, D.C. in November 1976 to consider in detail the government drug programs of the following six nations: Australia, Canada, Norway, Sweden, the United Kingdom and West Germany. Papers describing each of these countries are abstracted separately. In addition to these papers, the proceedings include an introduction, a ten-page bibliography, and transcripts of panel discussions on the following topics: reimbursement systems, financing methods, cost controls, program evaluation, formularies and utilization trends. A set of "researchable questions" is also included.

References, 0.

See abstracts 18, page 57; 97, page 58; 110, page 58; 149, page 60; 212, page 60; 257, page 62.

WERTHEIMER, ALBERT I., Editor. Public Health Service. Health Resources Administration. National Center for Health Services Research. DHEW Publication No. (HRA) 77-3186. Springfield, Virginia, National Technical Information Service, June 1977.

Report from the United Kingdom

257 National Health Service (NHS) schemes have existed in the British Isles since 1911; the present system was introduced in 1948 for England, Scotland, Wales and Northern Ireland. The Channel Isles and the Isle of Man also have health service systems. The service is available to all persons in the country, but visitors may not come specifically to obtain free treatment. Employees and employers make weekly contributions to the health service as part of the Social Service stamp. Patients may consult any general practitioner participating in the system. When a general practitioner refers a patient to a hospital, no charge is made for the treatment, maintenance or medicine. Outpatients and general practitioner patients pay a prescription charge of approximately $.32. Private patients in hospitals pay treatment costs, but receive their medication without additional charge; they may not obtain drugs through the NHS when not in the hospital.

More than 95 per cent of all prescriptions dispensed are covered by the NHS. Pharmacists must dispense in accordance with doctors' prescriptions. Pharmacists purchase pharmaceuticals through wholesalers or from manufacturers, and prices are controlled through the Voluntary Price Regulation Scheme of the Department of Health and the Association of the British Pharmaceutical Industry, based on each company's profit position. For generic drugs and other NHS prescriptions, payments to pharmacists are based on the average net price chargeable by the manufacturer or wholesaler.

If a generically prescribed drug is only available in proprietary form, the price reimbursed is based on the lowest priced proprietary product generally available. NHS hospitals generally purchase drugs on contract by Regional Health Authorities. The NHS Drug Tariff covers payments for drugs, appliances and chemical reagents, and specifies the quality of drugs to be supplied.

In sum, pharmacists are paid monthly, (1) the wholesale cost of drugs and appliances, (2) a container allowance of approximately $.03 per prescription, (3) a professional fee of approximately $.40, which varies by type of prescription dispensed, and (4) an on-cost allowance of 10.5 per cent of the wholesale cost of drugs and appliances dispensed. Additional payments are made for the provision of oxygen therapy equipment, after hours and holiday services and pharmacy services in rural areas. Rates are reviewed monthly. Pharmacists submit prescriptions monthly to a pricing bureau for processing and payment; computer handling of these tasks is being investigated. Details of profit and notional salary (total value of the proprietor to his or her business) calculations are offered; these factors affect payment rates to pharmacists and the size of prescription discounts for quantity.

References, 0. *Key words:* Maximum allowable cost, patient cost sharing, reimbursement.

WHITTET, T.D. *In* Wertheimer, Albert I., Editor. *Proceedings of the International Conference on Drug and Pharmaceutical Services Reimbursement.* Public Health Service. Health Resources Administration. National Center for Health Services Research. DHEW Publication No. (HRA) 77-3186. Springfield, Virginia, National Technical Information Service, June 1977. Pages 85–103.

1976

Comparative Approaches to Cost Constraints in Pharmaceutical Benefits Programs

141

Lee discusses United States and European approaches to constraints on drug expenditures under public health programs. He suggests that third-party programs reinforce the physician's tendency to use high cost treatment options; for example, if only inpatient drugs are covered, the physician concerned with the patient's economic welfare will recommend hospitalization. It is illogical for public programs to encourage this kind of activity. Rising drug costs are due to world-wide increases in the costs of raw materials and labor. Productivity may be hampered by the time and expenditures required to meet federal regulations.

He presents European experiences in determining utilization and controlling drug use by patient cost sharing. Some countries exempt certain categories (for example, retirees) from copayment. He concludes that research and development must be encouraged and that each country's goals must include the optimization of quality and quantity of health care within available economic resources. He prefers constraints that will reinforce the competitive market system rather than those that involve coercion.

In a critique of Lee's remarks, Leif Schaumann suggests equitable distribution and accessibility of health care services as a national goal. He discusses the experience of the Scandinavian countries and the reliance on efficient centralized planning, and questions the usefulness of international expenditure comparisons because of problems of definition. He recommends limited price controls on retailers and concludes that because of the societal characteristics of the United States, pharmaceutical benefits are best expanded on a piecemeal basis to minimize economic, social, scientific and political consequences, and that foreign experiences have limited applicability to the United States.

T. Donald Rucker disputes Lee's explanation of drug industry pricing practices and suggests more careful consideration of overhead costs and price competition. He recommends the establishment of a national computerized drug record system to collect and analyze data on prescriptions initiated and dispensed. He questions the ability of market forces to effectively regulate drug prices. Government policy should include the cooperative development of a uniform cost accounting system.

References, not counted; footnotes used. *Key words:* Drug utilization review, patient cost sharing.

LEE, ARMISTEAD M. *In* Mitchell, Samuel A. and Link, Emery A., Editors. *Impact of Public Policy on Drug Innovation and Pricing.* Proceedings of the Third Seminar on Pharmaceutical Public Policy Issues, December, 1975. Washington, D.C., American University, 1976. Pages 115–170, 170–177, 177–189.

1975

Pharmaceutical Industry. Price Regulation Scheme Erroneously Based, Says OHE Report

14

The Office of Health Economics (founded by the Association of the British Pharmaceutical Industry in 1962) published a report in September 1975 which criticized the voluntary price regulation scheme under which the National Health Service negotiates drug prices with manufacturers. The report argues that the normal competitive market forces will satisfactorily determine prices and maintain production levels, but that the voluntary price regulation scheme is based on the assumption that these market forces do not exist and, further, that the Department of Health uses this erroneous assumption to justify bureaucratic price controls, a system which has brought drug prices to a "dangerously low level," thus discouraging innovation. The Director of the Office of Health Economics stated that price competition for pharmaceuticals is just as effective as in any other market, and that, therefore, the market success of a prescription drug is affected by its price relative to those of alternative drug products. The Office of Health Economics is sponsoring a study by the University of Edinburgh's Department of Business Studies to show that free market forces determine competitive prices and allocation of resources more effectively than do government controls.

References, 1.

ANONYMOUS. *Pharmaceutical Journal 215* (5834):210, September 6, 1975.

Economics of Institutional Pharmacy Services under National Health Insurance in Australia

35

The National Health Scheme, which includes a Universal Pharmaceutical Benefits Scheme, was introduced in Australia in the early 1950's. It is estimated that 90 per cent of all outpatient prescription drugs are provided under the Pharmaceutical Benefits Scheme today. Governmental control over drug costs and the provision of pharmacy services are discussed. For each prescription dispensed, all community pharmacists are reimbursed on the basis of a "30 per cent loading on the wholesale price of drugs" in addition to a professional fee, which is negotiated between the Pharmacy Guild and the government. The fee-for-service system helps to ensure that a pharmacist is adequately compensated for increased workloads. Acquisition costs are negotiated between the Australian Minister for Health and the drug manufacturers. The use of a national formulary provides additional control over the drug manufacturers and over the prices for the drugs.

The method of reimbursement of public institutions for the cost of pharmaceutical services under the National Health Scheme is negotiated between the federal Minister for Health and the respective state ministers. The official policy of the federal government is to finance the costs of benefit drugs which are available in community practice; however, in effect, the government reimburses institutions for the costs of all drugs. Figures on the growth in demand for institutional services and the attendant costs of pharmaceutical services are presented. Several shortcomings of the present system of institutional reimbursement are outlined. A recently passed Health Insurance Act included the provision for a cost sharing agreement between the federal and state governments to equally finance hospital expenses, including the cost of pharmaceutical services. While the new system does improve the system of hospital financing, several questions about the methods in which the cost of pharmaceutical services is controlled are raised. The establishment of an Australian Pharmaceutical Commission is proposed and its prospective responsibilities are outlined.

References, 2. *Key words:* Formularies, inpatient settings.

BROOKS, GEOFFREY E.; and KNAPP, DAVID A. *American Journal of Hospital Pharmacy 32 (10)*:1018–1022, October 1975.

Pharmacy and the Health Maintenance Organization—The British Experience

37

This paper explores reasons why British pharmacists oppose the location of a pharmacy service in National Health Service (NHS) health centers, i.e. "on-site" location, in favor of the continuance of the present system of neighborhood pharmacies.

The position of the pharmacists is threefold: that there should be no on-site service if there are existing pharmacies convenient to the health center, that access to NHS dispensing contracts should be limited, since unlimited entry would threaten the economic viability of many small volume pharmacies, and that pharmacists should not be permitted to move into an area served by a health center if there are an adequate number of neighborhood pharmacies in the area. In 1968, legislation was passed that prohibited the employment of pharmacists by government authorities to serve in an NHS center, thereby reversing the provision contained in 1946 legislation which had been opposed by the pharmacists. No legislation has been passed to limit entry into NHS contracts.

Pharmacists argue that the system of neighborhood pharmacies must be preserved for three reasons: (1) the neighborhood pharmacist is a valuable source of health information to his patrons, (2) the neighborhood pharmacy is conveniently located for its customers, and (3) the neighborhood pharmacy is a British tradition. Several surveys which support or do not support the contention that pharmacists are valuable as drug advisors are extensively discussed, with the conclusion being drawn that it is not a valid argument for maintaining neighborhood pharmacies. The claim of convenience is discounted, since a patient must return to the physician, who is located at the health center, in order to obtain each prescription refill. A discussion on what advantages on-site location would offer the pharmacist centers around the opportunities for obtaining increased professional status by becoming a more participatory member of the health care team.

References, 32. *Key words:* Direct provision.

BUSH, PATRICIA J.; and WERTHEIMER, ALBERT I. *Journal of the American Pharmaceutical Association NS15 (12)*:691–695, 704, December 1975.

The United States and International Drug Regulatory Approaches

96

National drug use and price regulatory systems reflect a country's political, social, historical and cultural traditions, as well as the philosophies of the medical and pharmaceutical professions. For example, in England, the regulatory authority, a small review committee, works effectively with the assistance of outside experts. In the United States, in contrast, the FDA is a large, reserved, bureaucratic "policing" agency. There is also a difference in the type of public scrutiny; a discussion in England's House of Commons reveals a different attitude than hostile questioning by a Congressional committee. A consequence is that the British system is more flexible and responsive to the public interest in the matter of marketing new medicines. It is important to note, however, that the British system, based on centuries of tradition, could not be satisfactorily transplanted to the United States, where different traditional views of the roles of government and the pharmaceutical industry prevail. In the United States, regulation is based on product registration and the maintenance of drug quality. With the implementation of the Maximum Allowable Cost (MAC) program for federally purchased drugs, standards will be set to develop a list of interchangeable products with maximum reimbursement levels. This oversight of medical costs represents a new area of concern for the United States regulatory system, but is well established in Europe where every major country (except Switzerland) has some form of state reimbursement for drug expenditures.

In Canada, all citizens are covered by a medical plan which may or may not include drugs, depending on the province. The provinces are involved in product selection and have some form of substitution legislation. One plan maintains a formulary and participating pharmacists may substitute interchangeable products so long as the price of the dispensed product is lower. A national formulary plan, with province-by-province application, is being developed and will include acceptable prices which are expected to be sufficient to provide economic incentive for innovative drug manufacturers.

The voluntary price regulation scheme in England and the price regulatory system in France also consider economic incentives, but the British system has led to prices generally lower than in other European countries, which may have detrimental effects on the pharmaceutical industry. The import and sale of drugs within the European Economic Community (Common Market) are complicated by varying tariffs, registration and product test requirements, and other legislation. Some countries (until recently including the United States) will not accept clinical tests done in other countries as a basis for product approval. National formulas for retail sales prices also vary, and some fail to consider the research and development expenses of the originator, costs not borne by imitators. There is also difficulty in separating scientific from political judgment, a distinction that must be maintained if more uniform international standards and regulations are to be effective.

References, 5. *Key words:* Maximum allowable cost.

HELFAND, WILLIAM H. *Journal of the American Pharmaceutical Association NS15* (12):702–704, December 1975.

Community Pharmacy. Pharmacy and the National Health Service. Contractors' Attitudes

114

A 1972 survey of chemist contractors revealed general dissatisfaction with the National Health Service (NHS) contract remuneration, but little understanding of the philosophy behind it. Questionnaires were sent to 1465 pharmacy owners concerning their satisfaction with contract remuneration and terms of service. There were 821 representative usable responses. Over 74 per cent were "dissatisfied" or "very dissatisfied" with remuneration, and 41.3 per cent were unhappy with nonfinancial aspects. The most frequent comment concerned inadequate remuneration, particularly too low "on cost." The second most frequent criticism concerned ingredient cost reimbursement, particularly the level of automatic discounts. Other complaints included the reimbursement of pharmacists compared to other groups, rota and out-of-hours payments, lag behind inflation and return on capital. Contrary to expectation, contractors in large pharmacies were just as dissatisfied. Some contractors actually admitted ignorance about other terms of service. The biggest complaint was long hours. A number thought the total system was too inflexible and would have liked, for example, more leeway for professional judgment and initiative in providing service. Mistrust of the pricing bureau doubtless stems from faulty understanding of Drug Tariff procedures.

A more legitimate grievance is the requirement for a prescriber counter-signature on prescriptions that are clarified when dispensed. Other concerns were professional status, rota service organization, etc. Even allowing for the limitations of a postal survey, confusion and misconceptions about the contract were apparent in the comments made (and also reflected in the Linstead report). Few contractors saw remuneration as the composite yield of on-cost and professional fee. Revisions since 1972 may have assuaged some dissatisfaction. However, most contractors seem not to be aware that the "improvements" in distribution may represent a gain for some at the expense of others. Part of the problem is the system's complexity, but the Central NHS Committee definitely must upgrade education and the contractors' new association (Counterbalance), for improved communication certainly warrants support.

References, 23.

JONES, I.F. *The Pharmaceutical Journal 215* (*5831*):150–153, August 16, 1975.

Community Pharmacy. Pharmacy and the National Health Service. A Proposed New Charter for Pharmacy

115

Following a brief review of the philosophy of, and practical problems associated with, current remuneration practices, a "charter" is proposed to solve the imbalance in the current system of remuneration for the pharmacist under the British National Health Service (NHS).

The proposed method of remuneration would not be based on the number of prescriptions dispensed. Six "allocation" elements of NHS remuneration are suggested and discussed: (1) basic practice allowance, (2) seniority payments, (3) retirement benefit, (4) practice relocation fee to encourage equal distribution of pharmacists, (5) fee for late night and emergency dispensing services, and (6) holiday and vacation fees.

Fifteen advantages of the reallocation scheme are detailed, for example: (1) removal of the profit from the provision of the pharmaceutical service, (2) provision of a guaranteed income, (3) provision of a career structure for community pharmacists through the seniority payment component, and (4) provision for increased and more realistic planning of the NHS pharmaceutical service. Conditions which would need to be fulfilled by the pharmacist and the pharmacy are outlined. Several potential problems are raised, for example: (1) the difficulty in fairly distributing the workload, (2) the system might necessitate the registration of patients with a particular pharmacy, and (3) that of capital investment and the ownership of property, stock and fixture.

References, 22.

JONES, I.F. *The Pharmaceutical Journal 215* (5834):211–214, September 6, 1975.

Pharmacy and the National Health Service 1. Some Basic Issues

116 Provisions of the National Insurance Act of 1911, the forerunner of the current National Health Services (NHS) Act, are detailed in order to provide a historical and philosophical background to contract remuneration for chemist contractors under the NHS. Beginning in 1916, payments were made on a "cost price" tariff, in which the contractor received the estimated cost price for the drugs dispensed, plus a specified remuneration per prescription for professional services and overhead. This system has caused considerable frustration among chemists during its sixty-year history. Many of the same basic issues have been raised over the years: who should negotiate for the contractors? should threatened stoppage of services be used in bargaining? and should the number of pharmacies or NHS contracts be limited by statute? The chemists have historically bargained from a weak and disunited position and have reacted to external factors rather than controlled them. Historically, there has been no clear basis on which prescription remuneration has been founded. The dependence of pharmacies on NHS contracts for financial success has increased from 6 per cent in the late 1940's to 50 per cent in 1974. The decline in the number of pharmacies throughout the years is a trend which is expected to continue, and which will pose problems for the public, the profession and the State.

References, 34.

JONES, I.F.; and BOOTH, T.G. *The Pharmaceutical Journal 215* (5828):72–74, July 26, 1975.

Pharmacy and the National Health Service 2. Macro-Economic Aspects and Trends

117

Problems and issues associated with the remuneration system of the National Health Service (NHS), in which chemist contractors are paid on an item of service basis, are discussed. The number of prescriptions dispensed determines the amount of payment received under this system of remuneration. Since 1949, prescriptions have increased in number by 46 per cent and in total cost by 900 per cent, most of which is due to higher costs. Various cost figures (e.g., total cost per item, gross margin) are given for each year 1949–74. In real terms, the average on-cost plus professional fee increased only 10.7 per cent from 1949 to 1975. In real terms, a typical pharmacy owner received in 1974 approximately twice the gross profit per pharmacy received in 1949. This increase is due to a 46 per cent increase in the number of prescriptions dispensed and a 20 per cent decline in the number of pharmacies; it is not due to a greater unitary payment rate. For the same reason, the average total net profit per pharmacy (1964–70) has kept pace with the cost-of-living index. Chemist contractors have received a declining portion of NHS expenditures between 1953 and 1972. The number of prescriptions dispensed is analyzed by pharmacy size classification; in the future, it is expected that half of the pharmacies in England and Wales will be dispensing 75 per cent of the total number of prescriptions. The remaining 50 per cent of the pharmacies will be predominantly independently owned pharmacies, located primarily in local communities.

References, 21.

JONES, I.F.; and BOOTH, T.G. *The Pharmaceutical Journal 215* (5829):96–99, August 2, 1975.

A Quantitative Analysis of Antisubstitution Repeal

138

Prescription data from 20 Saskatchewan (Canada) pharmacies before and after the repeal of drug antisubstitution laws (January–June 1971 and January–June 1972) showed significant (0.05) increases in brand or generic substitution activity from 1.16 per cent to 3.08 per cent and in inpatient prescriptions, 4.61 per cent to 6.88 per cent. No significant differences were found in third-party prescriptions (16.54 per cent to 16.55 per cent) or in generic prescribing (9.80 per cent to 10.84 per cent).

In 1970, the Public Affairs Committee of the American Pharmaceutical Association sought repeal of state antisubstitution laws. Some states have responded, but not in sufficient numbers to examine the resulting patterns. Therefore, the study was undertaken in Canada, where Saskatchewan became the fourth province to repeal antisubstitution laws on July 1, 1971. Physicians may indicate "no substitutes," but otherwise pharmacists can generically substitute across trade names without a formulary. Average patient charges for all prescriptions and for substituted prescriptions decreased slightly between 1971 and 1972. The average charge for generic prescriptions did not change, but the average charge for brand name (nonsubstituted) prescriptions increased from $3.56 to $4.81. However, an examination of the prescriptions by unit price indicated a small price decrease over all prescriptions; a significant (0.05) price decrease for brand name (nonsubstituted) prescriptions (due, in part, to an increase in unit dispensed per prescription); a small price increase for generic prescriptions and a significant (0.05) price increase for substituted prescriptions (partly confounded by the great change in quantity dispensed per prescription). The 1972 unit price for substituted drugs remained lower than the unit price for brand name drugs, although it was higher than for generic drugs. Results cannot be extrapolated to the United States should there be repeal of antisubstitution laws, but such studies should provide insight into the economic effects.

References, 10.

KOTZAN, JEFFREY, A.; HUNTER, ROBERT, H.; and TINDALL, WILLIAM, N. *Medical Marketing and Media 10* (5):18–20, May 1975.

Experiences of the New Pharmacy System in Sweden

148 The Swedish pharmacy system since its consolidation under a government-sponsored company is described. A Medicines Act regulates the import, production and quality control of drugs. Pharmacies were regulated private enterprises until 1970, when the Apoteksbolaget AB (National Corporation of Swedish Pharmacies) was created to hold exlcusive right to the public distribution of drugs. It bought out all existing pharmacies and their owners became company employees. The company is responsible for ensuring the supply of drugs, disseminating drug research, providing optimal service, charging low and uniform prices that yield a reasonable return, and promoting information and statistics on drugs and drug use. Sweden's 25 counties, which are responsible for health care, cooperate in 7 health care regions. The company has 7 regional offices to service as liaison between its 683 pharmacies (it also has many other drug outlets) and has headquarters in Stockholm. Most pharmacies are small; a few very large. Sales were $500 million in 1974.

The staff is about 12,000 in total, 9,700 full-time and categorized as pharmacists, prescriptionists and technical assistants. To optimize staff productivity, which is up 14 per cent since 1972, doctors of pharmacy are generally chiefs of hospital pharmacies, pharmacists run the biggest community pharmacies and prescriptionists are in charge of small ones and do most of the dispensing. Ninety-six per cent of prescriptions are delivered immediately; the rest within 24 hours. There has been a 9 per cent increase in the number of pharmacies and 11 per cent have moved to improved locations.

Since Apoteksbolaget began wholesaling drugs in 1975, costs for this are probably lower than in any other country. Drug prices have increased, but less than prices in general. The organization's resources have been used to minimize local administrative burdens, e.g., by centralized, computerized payment of wages and invoicing. Apoteksbolaget is testing the use of computer terminals in several pharmacies to prepare labels and record information on prescribing patterns. The company has had a surplus each year except the first. It is just starting price negotiations with drug companies and expanding efforts at rational drug choice into outpatient care. Contrary to rumors, the system is succeeding. The cooperation of all institutions involved is necessary to attain the best health care.

References, 0.

LÖNNGREN, RUNE. *Journal of the American Pharmaceutical Association NS15* (7):379–381, 405, July 1975.

Pharmaceutical Services under the British National Health Service

206

Data on total drug and pharmacist costs and prescriptions dispensed under the British National Health Service (1949–1972) indicate that, while the volume of prescriptions declined with each increase in the amount of copayment required of patients, total expenditures continued to increase. Health insurance programs covering drugs should consider that, when copayments by patients are required, there is a tendency for physicians to increase the quantity of medication per prescription to offset the financial burden on their patients. Copayments in the British system increased from approximately 12¢ to 50¢ per item. Saskatchewan province (Canada) introduced the first government-sponsored, universal prescription drug plan in North America in 1975.

References, 1.

SCHNELL, B.R. *Drugs in Health Care* 2 (1):70–71, Winter 1975.

National Health Systems in Eight Countries

218

This publication describes the health care systems of Australia, Canada, the Federal Republic of Germany, France, The Netherlands, New Zealand, Sweden and the United Kingdom. For quick reference, the major characteristics of the health care system and health insurance system of each country are presented in tabular form. A complete chapter is then devoted to each country, in which details are explored. The following format is used in each chapter:

Background
Organization of health care delivery
- Physicians
  - General practitioners
  - Specialists
  - Hospital physicians
- Hospitals

Coverage
- Compulsory
- Voluntary
- Other

Benefits
- Medical
- Cash payments
- Maternity

Procedures for obtaining care
Role of private insurance
Financing
- Contributions
- Role of government
- Cost sharing

Reimbursement procedures
- General practitioners
- Specialists
- Hospitals
- Pharmaceuticals

A four page bibliography is included.

References, 0.

SIMANIS, JOSEPH G. United States Department of Health, Education, and Welfare. Social Security Administration. Office of Research and Statistics. DHEW Publication No. (SSA) 75-11924. Washington, D.C., U.S. Government Printing Office, January 1975.

Pharmacy in the United Kingdom

223 Britain's national drug insurance program, in effect since 1911, has made prescription drug benefits available since 1948, often at no charge to the recipient. The National Health Service is the largest single consumer of pharmaceuticals. Pharmacies operate under the auspices of the executive councils and pharmacists deal with them in order to provide services and receive payments. The executive councils also determine what the minimum hours for a pharmacy will be and they administer the Drug Testing Scheme, created to insure that those medicines and medical supplies which are dispensed are in accordance with the prescriptions for them. Pharmacies are selected by sampling technique and inspectors come into the premises to analyze the drugs. The pharmacist has an authority list of drugs for which payment is made, the *Drug Tariff,* which is updated regularly with new drugs, prices and quality standards. All those who practice pharmacy in Great Britain must belong to the Pharmaceutical Society, while at the same time there exists a National Pharmaceutical Union which represents private pharmacy owners and which is closely allied with the aforementioned organization. The changes occurring in general practice pharmacy may ultimately culminate in the nationalization of pharmacies in Great Britain, but whatever the results, they can serve as a role model for the United States in the shaping of pharmacy function.

References, 19. *Key words:* Formularies.

SMITH, MICKEY C. *Journal of the American Pharmaceutical Association NS15* (*12*):687–690, December 1975.

1974

PARCOST Comparative Drug Index

57 The objective of the PARCOST (prescriptions at reasonable cost) program is to assist the people of the province of Ontario in obtaining prescribed drug products of quality at reasonable cost by developing economies throughout the pharmaceutical industry and health professions. The program encourages fair competition and more efficient methods of distribution and utilization of pharmaceuticals made available through community pharmacies or hospitals.

The *Comparative Drug Index* lists prescription products by nature, strength and dosage form of the active therapeutic ingredient. Comparable products are listed according to trade and/or nonproprietary name and supplier or manufacturer, and are arranged in order of relative maximum cost. Categories of similar drugs are printed on color-coded pages. The *Index* is intended to serve as a guide to practitioners in the identification of quality products, to pharmacists for the stocking of comparable products, and to professional committees for the selection of products for use in hospitals. Interchangeable pharmaceutical products are noted. Prices represent pharmacist costs from wholesalers; patient costs include a dispensing fee not to exceed $2.20. A 1972 survey found that 57 per cent of the prescriptions written in the province were done so with the intention of reducing patient costs. This is taken to indicate confidence in the list of interchangeable drug products.

References, 0. *Key words:* Maximum allowable cost.

DRUG QUALITY AND THERAPEUTICS COMMITTEE. Seventh Edition. Ottawa, Canada, Ministry of Health, 1974.

National Health Service. Cost of Dispensing in the Pharmaceutical Services

170

The purpose of the study was to determine how much of the cost of the pharmaceutical services of the National Health Service (NHS) in England is due to the actual cost, i.e., manufacturer's, price of the drugs. The pharmaceutical contractors are paid by the regional executive council on a standard fee-for-services basis, while the pharmaceutical services of NHS hospitals negotiate drug prices more directly with the drug manufacturers.

Prescription price data were obtained from the Birmingham Pricing Bureau in December, 1972, and were expressed per unit medical manpower (i.e., prescriber). Analysis of the prescription price data showed that the NHS hospital price was only 60 per cent of the average payment made to the pharmaceutical contractors, if the latter amount included the pharmacist's professional fee, and 80 per cent if it did not. This difference, on the basis of the 60 per cent calculation, would amount to approximately 80 million (English) pounds annually (1972), of which 30 million (English) pounds would represent the difference in drug pricing and 50 million (English) pounds of the cost difference would represent the professional fee and running costs of the pharmaceutical service contractor. The difference in drug pricing results from the hospital practices of bulk purchasing of drugs and of purchasing by generic name. The running costs incurred by the pharmaceutical services contractor and not by the NHS hospital pharmaceutical services include the costs of providing drug quality control testing, maintaining a larger drug inventory, and remaining open for business for more hours.

In order to reduce the nationwide costs of pharmaceutical services, an alternative approach to dispensing drugs is suggested. The proposed system would include direct NHS-financed dispensaries attached to existing hospital outpatient departments or group practice centers with six or more family practitioners. Estimates of cost savings under the proposed system are presented.

References, 6. *Key words:* Direct provision.

OPIT, L.J.; and FARMER, R.D.T. *The Lancet:* *1* (7849):160, 162, February 2, 1974.

The Drug Business in the Context of Canadian Health Care Programs

204 Public health programs providing hospital and physician care are available to Canadians and are financed by tax revenues. Outpatient prescription drugs are thus the only health care expense the individual must absorb, and this has received a great deal of attention. At the retail level, much has been done to keep prescription drug prices from skyrocketing. In an effort to aid this measure, the federal government has attempted to encourage generic rather than brand name prescribing, and they have also intervened in the areas of quality control and retail pricing with a high degree of success. A scheme providing drug benefits is imminent, whether in conjunction with the Canadian government or as an independent venture on the part of some provinces. Perhaps a cost sharing health program on a federal-provincial level will be instituted.

References, 6.

RUDERMAN, A. PETER. *International Journal of Health Services* 4 (4):641–650, 1974.

Professional and Economic Bases for Pharmaceutical Services under the British National Health Service

227 The British National Health Service (NHS) system for reimbursing pharmacy owners is described. A committee of pharmacy representatives negotiates with the government for remuneration, to include: (1) container cost, negotiated after a cost survey, (2) ingredient cost, based on manufacturer or wholesale price, (3) overhead costs, based on a dispensing costs inquiry every few years in sample pharmacies that use work sampling analyses and financial records to compute a cost per prescription that is updated annually according to certain indices, (4) labor costs, based on data from the work sampling study, 6 staff categories and a negotiated proprietor's payment that considers hours worked, experience, etc., and (5) profit, a negotiated return on capital. Rising costs have been a serious concern since the 1950's. Data are presented which show changes in remuneration since 1948.

Administrative controls, not stringent by some United States standards, exert pressures toward "rational prescribing." A free *Prescriber's Journal* provides physicians with up-to-date information on drugs; a committee has been formed to evaluate drug effectiveness; the NHS annually sends each physician a month's comparison of his prescription quantities with national and local ones and contacts him if there is a large deviation. Placing the main burden for controlling drug utilization on physicians is possible because patients generally see only a single general practitioner or group practice and no refill prescriptions are given. Patient copayment for prescription drugs, introduced amidst great controversy (and with many exemptions) as a government economy measure, has also moderated demand.

Pharmacy owners may receive other compensation, including rural subsidies, rota duty payments for opening outside normal hours, "urgent" fees for emergency dispensing, out-of-pocket expenses, broken bulk payments for packages of drugs not normally stocked and fees for private prescriptions. Arguments through the years have centered on NHS reimbursement amounts and computation methods. A current dispute between the Pharmaceutical Society and the report of a Working Party representing several pharmacist groups concerns such matters as whether the remuneration system is too complicated and whether pharmacist advisory services can be isolated as a cost. General career discontent may be expressing itself in economic grievances.

References, 23. *Key words:* Drug utilization review, patient cost sharing.

SMITH, MICKEY C.; JONES, IAN; and BOOTH, T. GEOFFREY. *Drugs in Health Care 1* (2):59–73, Fall 1974.

Control of Drug Utilization in the Context of a National Health Service: The New Zealand System

250

The distinctive feature of the New Zealand medical system is the way in which payment for pharmaceuticals is arranged and aspects of this scheme are described. Advanced education in clinical pharmacology aids in assuring that effective drug usage will be maximized. In order for a drug to be prescribed it must appear in the *Drug Tariff*. What this means is that the basis of the Pharmaceutical Benefits scheme is the "limited list." Several other techniques of control have been implemented which concern themselves with safety and efficacy and they are: price determination made by the Department of Health, restrictions on duration and quantity of supply, restrictions on outlets to other than retail pharmacies, certain drugs recommended only by specialists, restrictions to approved indications, disciplinary measures, and initiation of the visiting practitioner scheme for purposes of advice or assistance. Furthermore, through this scheme, the Department of Health has been able to monitor adverse drug reactions and provide information about patterns of drug prescribing in New Zealand.

The New Zealand benefits scheme somewhat resembles the hospital formulary concept here in the United States, but features such as existing controls make it unique. Control over drug utilization rather than access to market appears to be the preferred alternative, and the New Zealand plan defines feasible methods to accomplish this. The future performances of this scheme and others like it will be of interest in order to recognize implications for the medical field.

References, 8. *Key words:* Drug utilization review, formularies.

WARDELL, WILLIAM M. *Clinical Pharmacology and Therapeutics 16* (3):585–594, September 1974.

1973

Trade Names or Proper Names?—A Problem for the Prescriber

106

A 1973 London symposium on prescribing by trade or generic name, attended by representatives of the pharmaceutical industry, pharmacists and medical practitioners, offered suggestions on the problem of drug substitution in the absence of therapeutic equivalence. In National Health Service Hospitals, pharmacists may substitute alternative brands of a drug product; this is thought to reduce both costs and processing time. Buying fewer drug products in bulk yielded savings amounting to approximately 1 per cent of the total National Health Service drug budget. Outside the hospital setting, substitution by pharmacists is not permitted. Variation in the effects of different formulations of the same drug has been found.

The pharmaceutical industry encourages brand name prescribing as a way of recovering research and development costs. Pharmacists prefer trade names because these drugs are more profitable and because there are differences between brands of drug products containing the same active ingredient. Also, pharmacists are unfamiliar with patient histories. Most general practitioners prescribe by brand name because they usually lack the time to study clinical trials reports and become familiar with drug products only through advertising. Researchers argue that generic names convey more information about active ingredients (especially important with combination antibiotics) and facilitate communication among medical personnel. Nurses request that whichever prescribing system is chosen, it be standardized. For therapeutic equivalence to be demonstrated, the correct quantity of the active ingredient and the fact that it reaches the site of action, must be established. It has been shown that formulation can affect absorption (bioavailability), especially with combination products. A National Pharmaceutical Laboratory to set drug standards was proposed.

References, 4. *Key words:* Inpatient settings.

HUSKISSON, E.C. *British Medical Journal* 4 (5886):225–228, October 27, 1973.

The Pharmaceutical Market and Prescription Drugs in the Federal Republic of Germany: Cross-National Comparisons

205 This paper examines prescription drug costs, the pharmaceutical market as a whole, and drug consumption in the Federal Republic of Germany. Cross-national comparisons are made with several countries, although doing so poses obvious difficulties.

The consideration of various aspects of per prescription costs shows that generic prescribing is declining in popularity and that the Federal Republic of Germany leads other nations in the abundance of pharmaceutical preparations available on the domestic market. A characteristic of this nation is an abundance of both pharmaceutical firms and products, as well as a large investment in promotional expenditures. These promotional costs do not influence prices as they do here in the United States. Distribution patterns also influence drug costs. In the Federal Republic of Germany, drugs are channelled to the consumer through independent pharmacies, which results in a substantial markup that is even higher than in other countries. It is concluded that the total per capita drug consumption costs in the Federal Republic of Germany are affected largely by a higher level of utilization. However, because of the comparatively lower cost per item, the total costs are commensurate with the outlays of other countries mentioned. Those changes which may occur in the per prescription cost may ultimately prove to be the major factor in determining the total per capita costs for prescription drugs.

References, 53.

SCHICKE, R.K. *International Journal of Health Services* 3 (2):223–236, Spring 1973.

Drugs and Pharmacy Services under the British National Health Service

222

Despite limits on comparability, useful information was obtained from an investigation of pharmacy services under the British National Health Service (NHS). The report discusses elements of the NHS programs that could be adapted for use in public drug programs in the United States, such as pharmacist remuneration and attitudes toward reimbursement and drug utilization review procedures, and program administration and administrative research. It provides general information on the NHS and terms of pharmacy service. Appendices include lists of persons contacted and publications resulting from the NHS study. The report includes a five-page bibliography.

References, 63. *Key words:* Drug utilization review, reimbursement.

SMITH, MICKEY C. Final Report. Department of Health Care Administration. Social Security Administration Grant No. 56096. University, Mississippi, University of Mississippi, 1973.

Research Report. Paying the Pharmacist under the British National Health Service

228

The administrative mechanism used in England to remunerate pharmacists for their services is thoroughly discussed. The system handled 247 million prescriptions in 1971. The reimbursement situation in England differs from that of the United States in a number of ways, for example: (1) the larger number of prescriptions in the United States would create problems not encountered in Britain and (2) certain United States state and federal regulations, e.g., maintenance of prescriptions on file by the pharmacist, would prohibit the wholesale transfer of the current British system. The administrative organization and claims handling operations of the Joint Pricing Committee and the regional pricing bureaux are described in detail. The timing and method of calculation of payment to the pharmacist by his local Executive Council is explained.

The four components of the prescription payment are: (1) net price of drug dispensed, which is determined by negotiation, (2) a professional fee for each prescription, (3) an "on-cost" allowance and (4) a container allowance. The profit for the pharmacist is included in the professional fee and "on-cost" allowance components. Surveys are conducted throughout England and Wales every three years to determine average overhead and labor costs for pharmacists, in order to calculate, respectively, the "on-cost" allowance and the professional fee. The system includes a copayment mechanism, in which a flat amount (20 pence in 1973) per prescription is paid by the patient. About half of all patients are exempted, for a variety of reasons, from the copayment. The copayment mechanism was reintroduced in 1968, after which there was a 7 per cent reduction in the number of prescriptions dispensed in the following twelve-month period. Computers are not used in claims processing, since automation cannot be economically justified due to the low administrative costs of the present system. Utilization review is manually performed, thus limiting the number of innovations which could be introduced to improve its sophistication. Both physicians and pharmacists are checked periodically to guard against prescribing and processing abuses.

References, 20. *Key words:* Drug utilization review, patient cost sharing.

SMITH, MICKEY C.; JONES, IAN; and BOOTH, T. GEOFFREY. *Inquiry 10* (3):57–64, September 1973.

1971

Pharmacy in a New Age

39

This publication discusses the historical background of the pharmacy profession in Canada, industrial pharmacy development, wholesale distribution of drugs, retail merchandising practices, nonmedical use of drugs, consumer protection, trends in modern health care, the role of the pharmacist and the pharmacist's assistant, pharmacy outlets, pharmacy manpower and pharmaceutical education in Canada, and the Canadian Pharmaceutical Association. Chapter 9, "Trends in Modern Health Care," discusses health insurance in Canada, several third-party drug programs, government and special drug programs, reimbursement policies, and administrative controls on third-party drug programs. A 63-page appendix deals with major research projects, presents additional tables and data and provides information on the provision of after hours pharmacy services, drug utilization review and control, and the interdisciplinary approach to drug distribution and utilization in hospitals and community or regional health centers.

References, not counted; footnotes used. *Key words:* Drug utilization review, reimbursement.

CANADIAN PHARMACEUTICAL ASSOCIATION. Commission on Pharmaceutical Services. Toronto, The Association, 1971.

1970

Drug Patents, Compulsory Licenses, Prices and Innovation

68

The United States patent and licensing provisions and similar laws in other countries, especially the United Kingdom, are reviewed. Special requirements for inventions relating to food and medicine are noted. Government hearings on patent protection and proposals to reduce patent terms on drugs from 17 to 3 years are discussed. The publication examines compulsory licensing and its relationship to market forces. Investment in research and development increases when there is a chance of realizing a new product that will be protected from unlicensed imitations for a period of time sufficient to recoup investment funds. The average research and development time is 8 years for a new product, and is increasing as government drug clearance and approval requirements become more stringent. A 1962 survey of 30 corporations found that 25 of them allocate 15–75 per cent more funds to research and development than they will if there were no prospect of obtaining full-term patents. Cases illustrating the positive and negative effects of compulsory licensing are presented. It was noted that the tendency of government agencies to take title to inventions arising from federally-funded research is discouraging to potential researchers. The publication suggests that charges of excessive profits in the pharmaceutical industry are unjustified.

References, 47.

A commentary by Frederick M. Scherer suggests that Forman is affected by "subjective perception." Scherer discusses his own survey (around 1959) of 91 American corporations which found that 52 per cent of them said that their research and development progress would be unaffected by compulsory licensing. He argues that the patent system slows innovation, as do image advantages and factors such as managerial experience or unique distribution channels. He proposes the compulsory licensing of drug patents, beginning three years after FDA approval of full-scale introduction of the product on the market.

References, 0.

A commentary by William W. Eaton suggests that the patent system stimulates invention and creativity and that widespread compulsory licensing will destroy the basics of the patent system. Eaton says that the drug industry and the medical profession should work together to provide information to the public about the drug scene.

References, 0.

A commentary by Leonard G. Schifrin suggests that prices are reasonable if they cover the costs of efficiently bringing forth products and making them available to consumers, if these prices also provide a profit level that justifies investment and risk-taking in drug innovation and manufacture. Schifrin endorses the three-year exclusivity period followed by compulsory licensing.

References, 0.

A commentary by Rosalind Schulman discusses the need for more flexibility in licensing and for the collection and analysis of relevant statistics. She offers data on products marketed, on company profits and on return on investment for the drug industry versus all manufacturing.

References, 3.

FORMAN, HOWARD I. *In* Cooper, Joseph D., Editor. *Economics of Drug Innovation*. Proceedings of the First Seminar on Economics of Pharmaceutical Innovation, April 1969. Washington, D.C., American University, 1970. Pages 177–198.

National Health Program Survey of Eight European Countries

176

This article surveys the health care programs of Belgium, Denmark, France, Germany, Italy, Spain, Sweden and the United Kingdom, with the assistance of Pharmaceutical Manufacturers Association counterparts, to obtain information that might serve as guidelines for United States legislators and administrators involved with national health insurance programs. It discusses, for each country: the legal basis for and history of the health care program; the program's administration, financing, coverage and benefits; the pharmaceutical component of the program (including government controls, product selection by physicians, place of purchase, copayments, drug program supervision and control, number of products per prescription and refillability); reimbursement procedures for physicians, pharmacies, or manufacturers; and trends and their potential impact on industry. Some European programs are financed by general revenues, some by government-controlled insurance, some by a combination and some by autonomous insurance funds. The programs cover 80–100 per cent of the population. A list of source materials on each country's health care program is supplied.

References, 53. *Key words:* Patient cost sharing, reimbursement, substitution.

PHARMACEUTICAL MANUFACTURERS ASSOCIATION. Washington, D.C., The Association, 1970.

1969

The Cost of Drugs

5

The strong emotional reaction to the subject of drug costs ignores the fact that, according to the recent report of a subcommittee of the Public Expenditure Committee, costs rose from just 0.3 per cent to 0.5 per cent of New Zealand's gross national product between 1946–47 and 1967–68. The Walsh Committee pointed out the difficulties of determining whether good value is obtained for the money; but decreases in general hospital bed use and duration of stay in mental hospitals imply benefits from improved medical care. Even though the country can clearly afford its drugs, they are expensive enough to warrant concern with cost control.

There can be little argument with the Committee's recommendations that proper education in prescribing is basic and that there should be more facilities to ensure the purity and efficacy of domestic and imported drugs.

Some Committee suggestions, such as abolishing brand names and permitting hospital boards to purchase drugs patented in New Zealand from nonpatented sources, are too simplistic. Many factors are involved in drug efficacy. The branded products of reputable firms are subjected to quality control and drugs from nonpatented sources should at least have to submit evidence of their clinical effectiveness. A *British Medical Journal* editorial supported the retention of brand names. The House of Commons decided against abolishing them because of international trade implications and opposed disregarding patents in purchases for the National Health Service. Incidentally, lack of patent protection is considered responsible for the Italian drug industry's notable lack of innovation and high prices. The Public Expenditure Committee has recommended setting up an independent Medicines Commission to be responsible for the licensing of drugs to be sold in New Zealand, for providing information to doctors, conducting research and planning on drug control, and advising the government on medicines. Evolution is inevitable, but radical changes and bureaucratic burdens that could stifle a system that has served so well must be avoided.

References, 3. *Key words:* Patents and prices.

ANONYMOUS. *New Zealand Medical Journal 69* (440):33–34, January 1969.

Pharmaceutical Aspects of the Australian National Health Scheme

92

The Australian national health care plan, an extensive scheme for providing medicines in addition to other health care services to its citizenry, is discussed. Pharmaceutical Benefits, available to anyone with a prescription from a certified medical practitioner, represent the most expensive area of health care benefits provided by the government, since they are not connected with health insurance and approximately 80 per cent of the medication supplied is paid for under this scheme. To help standardize this scheme, the Department of Health issues a *Schedule of Pharmaceutical Benefits* which lists the drugs allowed under coverage and subdivides this list according to those which can be freely supplied, those which are restricted, and those which are chemicals for use in extemporaneous preparations. An additional feature of the *Schedule* is that it lists the maximum quantity to be prescribed at any one time, how often the prescription can be renewed, its price and a code indicating the approved manufacturer. Since calculations and clerical work are complex and tedious, billing and payments have been computerized and systematized so that pharmacists can be paid at the end of each month. Some abuse of the system has occurred, but there has been a minimum of complaints from health care professionals. While the cost of the program has increased from $15.4 million in 1951 to $104 million in 1967, the United States can still learn many valuable lessons in the initiation of plans for third-party payment of prescriptions from the Australians.

References, 0.

HALL, NATHAN A. *Journal of the American Pharmaceutical Association* NS9 (4):184–186, April 1969.

1968

A Comparison of General Drug Utilization in a Metropolitan Community with Utilization under a Drug Prepayment Plan

87

Differences in drug utilization between the prevalent out-of-pocket payment system and a pharmacy-sponsored prepayment system in the Windsor, Ontario area were studied to shed light on the economic and functional impact of suggestions for coping with the large and unevenly distributed drug expenditures of United States consumers. A probability sample of some 3,400 prescriptions dispensed by Windsor area drugstores in 1962–63 was compared with age-adjusted utilization data under Prescription Services, Inc. (PSI), a program paying charges above a 35¢ deductible for out-of-hospital prescriptions.

The hypotheses tested were: (1) there are significant differences in utilization between the two systems; (2) drug prices are higher under the supplier controlled form of prescription payment; (3) financial factors in the community payment system produce an unmet need for drugs; and (4) patient influence has little effect on physician prescribing patterns in the prepayment plan. Hypotheses (1) and (2) were affirmed. Per capita, there were 2.19 prescriptions costing $8.29, or a mean prescription price of $3.78. The PSI subscriber rate was 4.20 prescriptions at a mean cost of $3.96 and $16.64 in annual expenditures. PSI rates applied to the total community would have increased costs about $1.6 million, 82 per cent for more medication and 18 per cent for higher prescription prices due to the $1.90 PSI minimum reimbursement and a 10 per cent reduction in the amount of medication dispensed per prescription. This contrasts with significant economies effected by the Group Health Cooperative of Seattle, Washington, which is organized so as to benefit from bulk purchasing, generic prescribing, a tight drug formulary, and nonprofit status.

Hypothesis (3) was tested by comparing utilization by demographic group and therapeutic class and analyzing the delay in dispensing prescriptions; hypothesis (4) by comparing physicians' prescribing patterns by type of practice, age and income. In brief, the data seemed to validate hypothesis (3), because the low-income widowed group had the greatest increase in utilization under PSI and single adults the smallest change; utilization by family increased with size under PSI only, the few prescriptions dispensed after 48 hours were generally costly ones, and greatest differential utilization rates under PSI correlated with therapeutic classes the patient could view as least serious. Findings bearing on the fourth hypothesis were mixed. There was little evidence of impact on prescribing patterns due to drug prepayment, but the more vulnerable general practitioners, young and old physicians and low-income ones, prescribed significantly more anti-infectives, psychotropics and amphetamines under PSI. Unmet need appears to warrant a change in financing drug delivery, but this must be accompanied by organizational change to reduce drug costs by rationalizing medical care services. Social, social-psychological and political efficiency should also be considered.

References, 17. *Key words:* Direct provision.

GREENLICK, MERWYN R.; and DARSKY, BENJAMIN J. *American Journal of Public Health* 58 (*11*):2121–2136, November 1968.

Current American and Foreign Programs

240 As part of the HEW Task Force on Prescription Drugs project, 6 federal, 10 state, 6 private and 13 foreign drug programs were reviewed. Each program is described in terms of its administration, eligibility requirements, benefits, reimbursement methods, cost controls and other regulations, and drug lists or formularies. Special characteristics of the retail pharmacy systems and drug industries are discussed for the foreign programs.

Federal programs include Department of Defense, Medicare, Military Medicare, Office of Economic Opportunity, Public Health Service and Veterans Administration; private programs include Prepaid Prescription Plans, PAID Prescriptions, United Mine Workers, Group Health Cooperative of Puget Sound, Kaiser Foundation Health Plan and Blue Cross Prepaid Prescription Program. Federal programs provide outpatient prescription drugs under several schemes, 31 states (in 1968) include some form of payment for drugs under Medicaid, and the number of private insurance plans covering outpatient prescription drug costs has increased markedly over the last few years. Some features of these drug cost programs may not be directly applicable to a national health program because of different population characteristics. There are 40 tables and 38 figures.

References, not counted; footnotes used. *Key words:* Formularies, reimbursement.

TASK FORCE ON PRESCRIPTION DRUGS. Background Papers. Office of the Secretary. United States Department of Health, Education, and Welfare. Washington, D.C., United States Government Printing Office, 1968.

1967

Drug Costs under Hospital Insurance

121

Pharmaceutical costs under hospital insurance plans, which include pharmaceutical benefits of ten Canadian provinces, were analyzed for the period 1961–65. A total of 99.3 per cent of Canada's population is covered by basic hospital insurance. The total cost of drugs in Canada for the five-year period increased from $29.6 million to $41.1 million, an increase of 38.6 per cent. The insured population increased during this period by 8.9 per cent. The cost of drugs as a percentage of total operating expenses of hospital insurance during this period decreased by 0.4 per cent. The national average cost of drugs on a per capita basis increased 24.5 per cent, from $1.63 to $2.03. No evidence was obtained to indicate that physicians were restricted in their choice of drugs due to economic factors.

References, 0. *Key words:* Inpatient settings.

KELLY, A.D. *Canadian Medical Association Journal 97* (8):425–427, August 19, 1967.

1962

Ironic Contrast: United States and Union of Soviet Socialist Republics Drug Industries

20

In both the Soviet Union and the United States, criticism is often leveled against four aspects of the country's pharmaceutical system: (1) the social and economic costs of promotion, (2) the role of research laboratories, (3) problems of brand differentiation and quality control, and (4) the relationship of the producer to the consumer. The specific criticisms within each general area are often reversed, a reflection of the differing economic systems of each nation. One major criticism of the American pharmaceutical industry is the high cost of promoting drugs, in part due to the practice of promoting brand and company names. One solution proposed to lower drug costs in the United States is to reduce promotional activity to simple announcements of new drugs and to eliminate the promotional activities of detail men. In the Soviet Union such a system has proved to be unsatisfactory, as physicians do not take the initiative or time to read the pharmaceutical literature. Soviet physicians are consequently criticized for not replacing old-fashioned drugs with newer, better ones. In the Soviet Union, pharmacy representatives are now sent to physicians to inform them of the drugs available. The closeness of the research and production functions within the United States drug industry and the separation of these functions in the Soviet Union are criticized by persons in each country.

In the Soviet Union, the institutional arrangements have resulted in problems of communication between research and production institutes and in bureaucratic delays between testing, evaluation and production. In the United States, however, the lag time between governmental approval and drug availability is usually nonexistent. Critics within the Soviet Union also criticize their drug industry for its lack of quality control. Manufacturers in the Soviet Union are being encouraged to adopt trademarks for identification purposes by the consumers in lieu of a quality control inspection system. Selective shortages within the Soviet system seem to be partly related to the stockpiling within pharmacies of products with a price which includes a large "planned profit." In the United States, the system of manufacturer's profits, industry competition and brand name drugs has resulted in better pharmaceuticals, due to the responsibility placed upon each manufacturer, and to the availability of more drugs, some of which may be unprofitable to produce, but whose lack of profits can be "balanced" through the production of more profitable drugs. The author's purpose in making this comparative study is to urge that alternative solutions to existing problems within the United States drug industry be examined before being adopted.

References, 13.

BAUER, RAYMOND A.; and FIELD, MARK G. *Harvard Business Review* 40 (5):89–97, September–October 1962.

Cross-References

For further information on other countries, see:

ABSTRACT NUMBER	PAGE NUMBER	ABSTRACT NUMBER	PAGE NUMBER
9	123	66	56
43	54	160	29
64	54	234	43

IV

Experiences in Inpatient Settings

Although the focus of the bibliography is outpatient prescribing, several cost containment approaches have originated in hospital settings. Items in this chapter deal with inpatient settings. Key words: Inpatient settings.

1976

Hospital Formularies: Organizational Aspects and Supplementary Components

203

An examination of the nature of supplementary sections and organizational features of hospital formularies suggests that the formulary is not generally employed effectively to transmit drug information and regulations.

Documents used to guide or restrict prescribing and responses to a brief questionnaire were received in February to March 1976 from 44 teaching hospitals with at least 500 beds (out of a national sample of 164 hospitals contacted). Considering that the provision of therapeutic guidelines has long been recognized as a supplementary formulary function, it is disappointing that 18 per cent of the formularies were just drug lists. Almost another 22 per cent had few supporting sections. Slightly over half listed drug products both alphabetically and by pharmacologic-therapeutic classification. The principle of generic nomenclature was followed exclusively by 60 per cent and in mixed form by 20 per cent.

Although 80 per cent included a background section on formulary development and use, clear definitions of the formulary's purpose or other significant information often seemed to be lacking. Forty per cent had not been recently revised. A little over half the sample formularies devoted sections to prescribing regulations and technical aids of various kinds. The same percentage had provisions more or less effectively aimed at lowering drug costs. Other types of supporting sections appearing in smaller numbers of formularies and included information on pharmacy services, drug products, patient medical condition and hospital regulations. There was a marked lack of uniformity in formulary physical characteristics. Only about a third were conveniently portable or easily updated. Although nearly half had superior readability, many suffered from small type, weak impression or other format problems.

General patterns emerging from the study were frequent inconsistency in the scope of coverage and in numerous administrative aspects. It is unclear what led to abbreviated guidelines, but it is unlikely that other methods of controlling prescribing or total practitioner knowledge explain the variability.

References, 5.

RUCKER, T. DONALD; and VISCONTI, JAMES A. *American Journal of Hospital Pharmacy* 33 (9):912–917, September 1976.

1975

A Cost Effectiveness Comparison of a Pharmacist Using Three Methods for Identifying Possible Drug Related Problems

50

Adverse drug reactions affect 18–30 per cent of hospitalized patients and cost approximately $3 billion for treatment. The relative effectiveness of a pharmacist (and the cost involved) in identifying potential drug-related health problems was studied for six months in a 34-bed medical ward of male and female adults using patient drug profiles, rounds with physicians and reviews of the patients' charts. Drug-related problems were defined as interactions involving: drugs and disease, more than one drug, drugs and food, allergic reactions, dosage regimen errors and overdoses (drug toxicity). The pharmacist, assisted by a pharmacy professor and a teaching physician, judged a drug-related problem to be clinically significant if the attending physician had noted an adverse effect on the patient's chart and discontinued the drug treatment. A total of 243 possible drug-related problems were detected. Of 224 patients who were studied, 124 had possible drug-related problems. Drug-drug interaction accounted for 71.6 per cent of the possible problems, but only 1.1 per cent were clinically significant. It was found that 20.1 per cent of the patients had 3 or more possible drug-related problems; 44.6 per cent had none.

The pharmacist was most effective in identifying problems from drug profiles from the hospital pharmacy (68 per cent), but only 5 per cent of these problems were clinically significant. Attending rounds was the least effective way of identifying possible drug-related problems (36.2 per cent), but the most effective way of identifying those that were clinically significant (22.4 per cent). Effectiveness with chart reviews was 56.1 per cent for possible drug-related problems and 19.9 per cent for those that were clinically significant. Costs per problem were $1.06 for reviewing drug profiles, $5.38 for reviewing charts and $8.68 for attending rounds. Rounds, while expensive, established a rapport with physicians and kept the pharmacist abreast of current drug therapies. Reviewing records and charts detected problems that had already been dealt with, and information was found to be incomplete. Attending rounds, the pharmacist could prevent possible problems and assist in offering the best possible patient care. Patients with clinically significant drug-related problems required extended hospital stays. At an average cost per patient of $101 per day, the increased hospital costs for the patients studied were $5656. This should be compared with the cost of the possible drug-related problem detection methods.

References, 13. *Key words:* Drug utilization review.

DICK, M. LAWRENCE; WINSHIP, HENRY W. III; and WOOD, GEORGE C. *Drug Intelligence and Clinical Pharmacy* 9 (5):257–262, May 1975.

Drug Utilization in the Hospital: An Evaluation of Drug Costs

153

Cost data for nine common drug groups administered to 7423 general medical service inpatients (August 1, 1969—March 13, 1973) show that certain drug groups were responsible for a disproportionate share of hospital pharmacy costs. The average number of drugs administered to each patient was 8.04. The average annual cost of drugs for the nine index drug groups administered during the study period was $24,948, half the total drug costs for these patients. Demographic data on the patients were obtained from hospital admission forms. Data on drugs administered were recorded on special medication forms and processed by computer. Cost data were obtained from the hospital pharmacy and from state contracts.

The three most expensive index drug groups (six antimicrobial, four anti-inflammatory, two anticoagulant) accounted for 81 per cent of the total cost of all drug groups studied, but only 22 per cent of the total patient exposures to the drugs studied. The three least expensive drug groups (five analgesic, four antiarrhythmic, four sedative-tranquilizer) accounted for 11 per cent of the cost (and the lowest average per patient cost), and 62 per cent of the patient exposures. The other drug groups (three antihypertensive, three diuretic, three antacid) accounted for 8 per cent of the cost and 16 per cent of the patient exposures. Cost, utilization and dosage data are presented for each drug in these groups. Reducing the costs of the three most expensive drug groups studied by 10 per cent would result in an 8 per cent cost reduction over all drug groups. The utilization of some drugs declined during the study period when new drugs were introduced (some at higher costs and some at lower costs). Changes in dosage form also affected costs, as did drugs which required laboratory tests and frequent patient monitoring. Drug utilization review is recommended to assess both patient welfare and hospital expenditures.

References, 16.

MAY, FRANKLIN E.; STEWART, RONALD B.; and CLUFF, LEIGHTON E. *Drugs in Health Care* 2 (3):139–152, Summer 1975.

How Drugs Attain Formulary Listing

186

Three hundred and five hospitals in total (representing various regions and sizes) receiving Medicare funds were surveyed by questionnaire to determine formulary use (required by Medicare law) and the selection process for drugs included in the formulary. A total of 172 hospitals (56 per cent) returned the questionnaires. Despite Medicare requirements, 18 per cent of the hospitals did not have a formulary. The responses of the 141 hospitals that did have a formulary or drug list were analyzed by bed size (8 groups, from 6–24 beds to 500 and more beds). Seventy-three per cent operated with a formulary system—a formal selection and evaluation process; up to 27 per cent of the hospitals, therefore, may include drugs in the formulary with no evaluation. Eighty-nine per cent of the hospitals have their pharmacy and therapeutics committee approve the formulary. The committee usually has full responsibility for evaluating drugs considered for inclusion in the formulary. Written policies for approving drug inclusion in the formulary were found in 65 per cent of the hospitals. The amount of information required from physicians who request the inclusion of a drug in the formulary increases with hospital size. Most hospitals allow physicians to prescribe drugs which are not in the formulary. The number of factors used in evaluating drugs for inclusion increases with hospital size. Most hospitals revise their formularies one or more times a year. Data support the thesis that hospitals act effectively in selecting drugs for inclusion in formularies. Guidelines are suggested, such as establishing procedures for obtaining permission to use drugs not in the formulary, specifying information to be obtained in evaluating drugs, and indicating the information to be included in the formulary on each drug.

References, 4.

ROLANDS, THOMAS F.; and WILLIAMS, ROBERT B. *Hospitals* 49 (2):87–89, January 16, 1975.

Drug Usage Review and Inventory Analysis in Promoting Rational Parenteral Cephalosporin Therapy

220 The pharmacy and therapeutics committee of the Shands Teaching Hospital at the University of Florida formed a subcommittee to evaluate parenteral cephalosporins on the basis of inventory, cost and use data. The subcommittee rejected a request to add cephapirin to the hospitals's formulary because budgetary constraints precluded adding a drug that offered no significant advantages. It determined that cefazolin, which the subcommittee felt was preferred in most cases, and cephalothin, with which the medical staff had more experience, were the main drugs to be considered. It also agreed that cephalosporins were being overused for staphylococcal infections.

The pharmacy supplied data on expenditures for top dollar usage systemic antibiotics in 1973 and 1974, a comparison of the costs of cephalothin, cefazolin and cephapirin at different dosage regimens, and a classification of cephalothin and cefazolin orders. Relative costs varied with the dosage schedule used. The subcommittee concluded that cefazolin was often used in too high a dose (1 g rather than 500 mg) and at too frequent intervals (q 6 hr rather than q 8 hr) and that modifying this would be the most economical approach. Data and recommendations were presented to the full committee, which notified the medical staff (by a memorandum) that it would delete cephalothin from the formulary in 6 weeks. A decision to purchase cefazolin on bid lowered the price further.

Objections by some staff members and pharmaceutical company representatives brought the cephalosporin decision up for debate again. A review of the pharmacology of both drugs turned up articles suggesting that cephalothin may be less nephrotoxic and that it penetrates the eye. The committee modified its decision slightly to permit its use in opthalmologic and impaired renal function patients. The usage of cefazolin increased dramatically thereafter, and dosage regimens changed somewhat. Continual education has proved necessary, however. Factors that will have to be monitored in the future include the substitution of other antibiotics, trends in route of administration and related side effects, optimum storage possibilities, drug shortages, and changes in patient population.

References, 12. *Key words:* Drug utilization review.

SIMON, WAYNE A.; THOMPSON, LOUIS; CAMPBELL, STUART; and LANTOS, ROBERT L. *American Journal of Hospital Pharmacy 32 (11)*:1116–1121, November 1975.

Potential Economic Effects of a Brand Standardization Policy in a 1000-Bed Hospital

237

The potential economic effects of a brand standardization policy in a 1000-bed hospital utilizing a unit dose drug distribution system were examined. Fifty high-use, nonproprietary drugs available commercially were selected for study and their drug usage and drug inventory costs were compared under a formulary and nonformulary system. Drug usage cost was defined as the dollar value expended by the hospital in order to purchase the drugs administered, and drug inventory cost was defined as the dollar value of drug products being stored for use in the hospital pharmacy. For the fifty drugs under examination, the use of this brand standardization policy was found to yield potential savings of more than $35,000 for drug usage costs and in excess of $9,000 for drug inventory costs. As a result of this study, it was concluded that a brand standardization policy would lower drug usage and inventory costs, that it would reduce the quantity of inventory items, and that such a policy could be implemented with a minimum of difficulty.

References, 20.

SWIFT, ROBERT G.; and RYAN, MICHAEL R. *American Journal of Hospital Pharmacy 32 (12)*:1242–1250, December 1975.

1974

A Statistical Approach to Per Diem Pharmacy Pricing

24

A three-part per diem charge system for hospital pharmaceutical services, based on (1) a daily professional fee, (2) the per diem drug charge, and (3) the cost of drugs not covered by the per diem charge, was developed from the analysis of one month (Spring 1968) of nursing records of daily drug administration (5313 patient days) to the maternity and internal medicine services of a large midwestern teaching hospital and the alcoholic treatment unit of a small midwestern chronic care hospital. Distributions of drug costs per patient day showed means from 30¢ to $1.88 and standard deviations from 12¢ to

$7.00. The distributions were skewed, indicating that only a small proportion of total patient days are relatively expensive; in other words, relatively expensive drugs account for only a small proportion of total drug use (frequency polygons and analysis of variance results are presented). By excluding the relatively few higher-priced drugs, the great majority of drugs can be included in a per diem charge which will allow the hospital to recover costs efficiently without over- or undercharging patients more than 53¢ per patient day. The few expensive items should be charged directly to patients at invoice cost.

The per diem drug charge should be calculated by comparing mean and median per patient drug costs, excluding the most expensive drugs, for a sample of patient days and recalculating until the mean and median drug costs become close; this is taken as the per diem drug charge. The daily professional fee should be calculated by adding nondrug operating expenses, allowing for capital improvements, depreciation, etc., and dividing by the total number of patient days. Under this three-part statistical system, the majority of pharmacy charges are automatically calculated by the hospital business office from patients' admission and discharge dates. The pharmacy initiates charges for those few drugs not included in the per diem drug charge. Pharmacy and nursing personnel are thus freed from the considerable time spent on drug charging activities for more professional pursuits. Also, per diem charges to the patient would appear more directly related to professional services.

References, 12. *Key words:* Reimbursement.

BOWER, RICHARD M.; and HEPLER, CHARLES D. *American Journal of Hospital Pharmacy 31* (*12*):1179–1188, December 1974.

1973

Pharmacy Purchasing, Formularies and Prices Paid for Drugs: A Survey of Hospitals in Southern New York State

161 A survey of practices in hospital pharmacies was carried out in the southern counties of New York State with the cooperation of the American Hospital Service (AHS) in order to see to what extent the concept of "prudent buyer" was pertinent. Questionnaires were sent by mail to 154 hospitals affiliated with AHS and 125 returned responses. The major aspects discussed were formulary practice, market concentration among pharmaceutical suppliers to hospitals, and prices paid by hospitals for drugs.

Of the responding hospitals, 88 per cent had implemented the formulary concept and most kept it current. In over half of the hospitals, between 95–100 per cent of all prescriptions were based on formulary drugs; however, on the whole, the formulary had a varied effect on drug choice. There was also variation in the extent to which hospitals relied on any manufacturer as a drug supplier, although leaders were in evidence. Almost all noted a price advantage when dealing with manufacturers rather than wholesalers, in addition to other advantages. In measuring hospitals as "prudent buyers," hospitals were asked about the purchase of six cited drugs, according to brand specified, price paid and frequency of order. While the results show a wide variation in price, as well as in preference for generic vs. trade name drugs, a bias against generic drugs was evident. If generic drugs were tested for biological efficacy and quality as they are being done in Canada at minimal cost, there would be a greater willingness to purchase generically without the fear of loss of quality. Suggestions were also offered to improve the rationality of prescribing and purchasing, such as developing and improving formularies and using alternative drugs.

References, 10. *Key words:* Substitution.

MULLER, CHARLOTTE; and KRASNER, MELVIN. *American Journal of Hospital Pharmacy 30* (9):781–789, September 1973.

How Cost-Effective Are Generics?

258

Blue Cross called upon the Pennsylvania Insurance Commission (PIC) to study cost differences between generic and brand name drugs. A study was designed to determine the validity of PIC's conclusion that if generic prescribing were the norm, a saving of between 60–95 per cent would result. Also, it would determine the effect of this saving on the payment for drugs to hospitals.

A stratified sample, which included 20 per cent of the 95 hospitals in Western Pennsylvania, was classified into five categories according to daily census. A tabulation was then made of each prescription filled by the pharmacy service within a 24-hour period. Data included the drug's name, strength, quantity and cost to the hospital. In all hospitals included in the study, more than half of the drugs prescribed were purchased at the lowest *Red Book* price. Of the drugs prescribed, 25 per cent were obtained at prices below the *Red Book* figure. It appears that, as a result of bulk purchase or membership in a group purchasing plan, hospital pharmacies can purchase drugs at a cost lower than the lowest *Red Book* price, and thus save $700,000 above savings secured through *Red Book* purchasing. Savings through the purchase of generic equivalents saves only 3.5 per cent of total drug costs, or about $600,000 for the area. This falls well below the projected 60–95 per cent savings. Thus, requiring generic prescribing would have little effect. The only way to secure a substantial decrease in drug costs to hospitals would be through a national quality testing program which would cut $42 million. A revision of the inefficient drug purchasing plans already existing would also be helpful.

References, 4.

WOLFE, HARVEY. *Hospitals* 47 (9):100, 104, 106, 108, May 1, 1973.

1971

Physicians' Prescribing Habits. Effects of Medicare

166

The effect of third-party payments for prescription drugs on physicians' prescribing habits was studied in a 540-bed teaching hospital for five disease categories with pre-Medicare and Medicare patients. No significant difference in average drug costs was found.

Records of patients aged 65 or older were compared for January 1–June 1, 1966 (pre-Medicare) and January 1–June 1, 1970 (Medicare) to determine differences in prescribed drugs for neoplasm, nervous and sense organ, circulatory, digestive and genitourinary diseases in terms of average days of hospital stay, number of drugs used and average cost of drugs. Fifty patients selected at random were included in each disease category under each time period. The days of stay and number of drugs used were obtained from hospital records. Drug costs were obtained from invoices current at the time of the prescription.

A table presents data for average days of stay, number of drugs and cost of drugs for each disease category (and for all diseases) for pre-Medicare and Medicare patients. Standard deviations, per cent change and values are included. Variation can be seen in most categories, but no differences were significant at the five per cent level. The findings do not support the frequent criticism that increased drug costs are due to an increase in the number of drugs prescribed, or to the prescribing of more expensive drugs under third-party payment plans such as Medicare.

References, 3. *Key words:* Drug utilization review.

NITHMAN, CHARLES J.; PARKHURST, YALE E.; and SOMMERS, E. BLANCHE. *Journal of the American Medical Association 217* (5):585–587, August 2, 1971.

1969

Administrative Profiles. Cost of Pharmacy Services

3

The major portion of pharmacy service expenses are for supplies rather than salaries and these expenses appear to be relatively stable among similar hospital groupings. For those hospitals with between 50 and 74 beds, the median cost for supplies averaged $2.10. This cost was $2.39 for those hospitals with 150 to 199 beds. Of those hospitals with 100 or more beds, 95.9 per cent employed a pharmacist. For hospitals with fewer than 100 beds, pharmacy salary expenditures were lower. This was due to the fact that hospitals in that category employ only a part-time pharmacist.

References, 0.

ANONYMOUS. *Hospitals 43 (16)*:28, March 16, 1969.

A Fee-Per-Patient-Per-Day Basis for Delivering Pharmaceutical Services to an Institution

99

Franchising pharmacy services to small hospitals on a fee-per-patient-per-day basis provides better control of drug costs and more complete pharmacy services. The experiences of the Hennessy pharmacy in extending services to Saratoga (Michigan) General Hospital are described. In 1954, Hennessy supplied professional staff to the 75-bed facility for a fee of $1000 per month, and controlled the storage and dispensing of drugs by placing all medical orders on prescription. A pharmacy and therapeutics committee was established to improve cooperation with physicians and a program to explain new pharmacy procedures to the nursing staff was implemented. A pharmacy manual, forms for recording the use of narcotics and new patient medication forms were developed. Business procedures were also simplified. The problem of providing pharmaceutical services beyond the 40-hour workweek was handled by making a pharmacist available at 8:00 p.m. to process additional orders. A pharmacist was always on call in emergencies. In 1968, a $1.00 fee-per-patient-per-day plan was proposed to the hospital (then 210 beds) based on the success of the Pontiac Plan (Pontiac, Michigan, General Hospital) in which a group of private physicians, through a corporation, took over the administration of the emergency room. A parallel was seen with the hospital pharmacy service and the approach has provided complete, continuous pharmacy service at a reasonable cost.

References, 0. *Key words:* Reimbursement.

HENNESSY, WILLIAM B. *Journal of the American Pharmaceutical Association NS9 (11)*:561–562, November 1969.

1966

The Financial Effects of Formularies in Hospitals

189

The financial performance of pharmacies in 24 nonteaching Chicago hospitals was assessed through two measures: cost of drugs per inpatient day and the formulary inventory turnover rate. For the size of hospital studied (216 to 417 bed capacity) the data showed, paradoxically, that as formularies become more restrictive, the financial performance of the pharmacies tends to deteriorate. However, the data also showed that several other factors affect a pharmacy's financial performance: consent agreements, number of items stocked, frequency of trial of new drugs and hospital size. Consent agreements were associated with an increase in the inventory turnover rate and especially with a decrease in drug cost per inpatient day, thus leading to improved financial performance. Financial performance also improved as frequency of trial of new drugs decreased and as hospital size increased.

References, 3.

ROSNER, MARTIN, M. *American Journal of Hospital Pharmacy 23 (12)*:673–675, December 1966.

Cross-References

For further information on inpatient settings, see:

ABSTRACT NUMBER	PAGE NUMBER	ABSTRACT NUMBER	PAGE NUMBER
31	179	109	189
32	173	121	83
35	153	167	150
63	209	180	182
69	220	182	192
106	75	233	178

Section Two

Cost Containment Approaches in Outpatient Drug Programs

Chapters in this section deal primarily with specific approaches to controlling costs in drug programs.

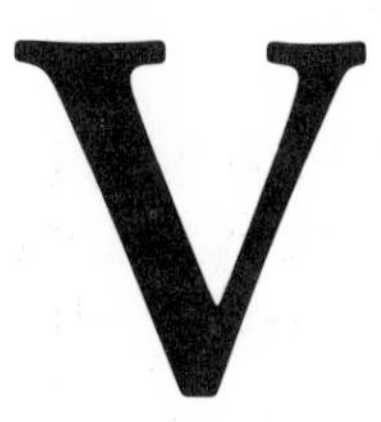

Patient Cost Sharing

One obvious method of reducing third party expenditures for benefits is to shift part of the cost to the patient via deductibles, coinsurance, and/or copayment.
Key words: Patient cost sharing.

1977

Coinsurance and the Demand for Physician Services: Four Years Later

209

A follow-up study on the effects of copayment on the demand for health care services under the Group Health Plan at Stanford (California) University found that utilization had remained fairly constant in the four years since the 1967 introduction of a 25 per cent copayment policy on all physician and outpatient ancillary services. The use of physician services in 1966 and 1968 (before and after the introduction of coinsurance) had been compared and a 24 per cent decline in demand for services noted.

The present study, undertaken to determine if copayment had a lasting impact, compared data for 1968 and 1972. Physician visits among the approximately 3500 subscribers were found to be 5.2 per capita in 1966, 3.9 in 1968 and 3.6 in 1972. Costs of physician services per capita rose 22 per cent from 1968 to 1972. Costs of lab tests rose about 24 per cent, costs of x-rays 57 per cent and costs of ancillary services almost 100 per cent. The use of x-ray and ancillary services per capita remained constant from 1968 to 1972, but lab tests rose from 3.1 in 1968 to 8.0 in 1972.

Data from a post-1967 group of subscribers, who joined the plan after coinsurance (thus never experiencing the "free" system), showed little difference in their demand for medical services from the pre-1967 group. Enrollment figures for nonprofessional staff subscribers dropped 36 per cent from 1966 to 1972; apparently, the 25 per cent copayment made the plan unsuitable for lower-income families.

References, 2.

See abstract 210, page 102.

SCITOVSKY, ANNE A.; and McCALL, NELDA. *Social Security Bulletin 40* (5):19–27, May 1977.

1975

Cost Sharing and Prior Authorization Effects on Medicaid Services in California: Part I. The Beneficiaries' Reactions

101 During the period from January 1972 to June 1973, a patient cost sharing experiment was conducted within the California Medi-Cal Program as a means of cost containment. A sample of beneficiaries was required to pay a $1.00 copayment for each doctor visit and a 50¢ copayment for each prescription for a maximum of two prescriptions per month. The underlying assumptions of this study were: (1) overuse is a major cause of increased costs of the program, and (2) this overuse can be controlled by the patient's decision as to whether or not he can afford the copayment. In this way the program was placing a share of the burden on the beneficiary to decide the need for medical care and the validity of services.

Approximately 30 per cent of the Medi-Cal beneficiaries were designated copayers. An interview survey was made of those beneficiaries who participated throughout the 18 months of the experiment. It was found that most had poor knowledge of the program and tended to confuse copayment with another restriction of the program known as concurrent constraint, or prior authorization for certain classes of services. With respect to physician visits, approximately 75 per cent of the respondents said that the copayment was collected at the time of the visit. Regarding prescription drugs, 12 per cent of the respondents said that they paid nothing. Most thought that the copayment had not affected their health care; however 17 per cent felt that it had reduced the care available to them, and these were primarily members of households with high medical needs. Only 12 per cent of the beneficiaries reported that the prescription copayment had kept them from getting prescribed drugs; but 39 percent of those "affected by copayment" said that it had affected their obtaining prescription drugs.

References, 7.

HOPKINS, CARL E.; ROEMER, MILTON I.; PROCTER, DONALD M.; GARTSIDE, FOLINE; LUBITZ, JAMES; GARDNER, GERALD A.; and MOSER, MARC. *Medical Care 13* (7):582–594, July 1975.

Cost Sharing and Prior Authorization Effects on Medicaid Services in California: Part II. The Providers' Reactions

102 Providers for the California Medicaid program were interviewed to determine their reaction to two new features of the program: (1) a copayment provision of $1.00 for each of the first two outpatient services, and (2) a limitation of services to two per month per individual without prior authorization by a Medi-Cal consultant for additional services and drug prescriptions. Four types of providers in urban and rural counties were surveyed: private physicians, hospital outpatient departments, pharmacies and nursing homes. Interviews were conducted during the last two months of the 18-month experiment.

Physicians, pharmacists and nursing homes thought copayment was not a hardship on their patients. Collection of the copayment was generally not a problem. Four of the 15 hospital outpatient departments surveyed did not attempt to collect the copayment. Private and hospital physicians generally did not alter the treatment given to copayers. All providers expressed greater concern over problems created by the prior authorization requirements than by the copayment requirement. Criticism of the prior authorization program centered about the additional paperwork required, the delays necessitated in giving treatment and interference with the treatment of patients. Reactions to the copayment provision might have been stronger had that provision been introduced without the prior authorization requirement.

References, 1.

HOPKINS, CARL E.; ROEMER, MILTON I.; PROCTER, DONALD M.; GARTSIDE, FOLINE; LUBITZ, JAMES; GARDNER, GERALD A.; and MOSER, MARC. *Medical Care 13* (*8*):643–647, August 1975.

Copayments for Ambulatory Care: Penny-Wise and Pound-Foolish

185

From January 1, 1972 until June 30, 1973, an experiment was conducted with California Medi-Cal patients where a $1.00 copayment was imposed for physician visits and a 50¢ copayment for prescription drugs. This copayment applied to the first two visits to a doctor in a given month and to the first two prescriptions in a given month. Data on rates of utilization were collected for a six-month period before the beginning date and for 12 months after the beginning date of January 1, 1972. There were at that time other administrative requirements in the program, such as prior authorization of certain services. These probably played some part in the experiment, although it is not known exactly what their role was.

It was found that following the start of copayment, the utilization rate of outpatient physician visits and other services associated with them showed a decline relative to the noncopayment group. After a brief lag, however, it was found that hospitalization rates among the copayment group rose to levels higher than those of the noncopayment sample. These rates more than offset any savings from the reduction of ambulatory service use rates. Higher hospitalization use rates suggest that financial deterrents to the excessive use of ambulatory services such as physician visits and prescription drugs by poor people are penny-wise and pound-foolish. This is presumably due to the neglect of earlier medical care because of the inhibiting effects of copayments.

References, 8.

ROEMER, MILTON I.; HOPKINS, CARL E.; CARR, LOCKWOOD; and GARTSIDE, FOLINE. *Medical Care 13* (*6*):457–466, June 1975.

Pharmaceutical Services under the British National Health Service

206

Data on total drug and pharmacist costs and prescriptions dispensed under the British National Health Service (1949–1972) indicate that while the volume of prescriptions declined with each increase in the amount of copayment required of patients, total expenditures continued to increase. Health insurance programs covering drugs should consider that when copayments by patients are required, there is a tendency for physicians to increase the quantity of medication per prescription to offset the financial burden on their patients. Copayments in the British system increased from approximately 12¢ to 50¢ per item. Saskatchewan province (Canada) introduced the first government-sponsored, universal prescription drug plan in North America in 1975.

References, 1.

SCHNELL, B.R. *Drugs in Health Care 2 (1)*:70–71, Winter 1975.

1974

Ambulatory Medicare Prescription Drug Study

140 A two-year pilot project is proposed in order to accumulate accurate data on drug costs for the elderly and to provide information on possible drug utilization patterns after passage of an outpatient drug program. PAID Prescriptions will provide comprehensive prescription drug coverage to a sample of Title XVIII patients in three California counties. Medicare patients participating in the study will be chosen by the Social Security Administration (SSA). All patients will receive all prescriptions from the 25,000 participating United States pharmacies for a $1 copayment, a 20 per cent copayment, or no copayment (control group). The recommended sample size is 1200 each for the experimental groups ($1 copayment and 20 per cent copayment) and 400 for the control group. Data will be collected for the middle six months of each year of the two-year study. Pharmacies submitting claims forms will be reimbursed on a cost-plus-dispensing-fee basis. Claims forms offer the following data: identification number, age, sex, date prescription dispensed, name of drug, dosage, quantity, price, number of days of therapy, pharmacy identification number, physician identification number and prescription number. Claims will be processed by computer and quarterly data will be provided to SSA on drug costs, utilization and the impact of the various copayment plans. Utilization review activities differ among the three counties in the study; data on cost and quality of drug therapy will be monitored.

References, not counted; footnotes used. *Key words:* Drug utilization review.

LAVENTURIER, MARC F. Social Security Administration Proposal. Burlingame, California, PAID Prescriptions, Incorporated, 1974.

1973

Changes in Prescription Drug Utilization after the Introduction of a Prepaid Drug Insurance Program

251 A prepaid drug prescription plan for United Auto Workers members and dependents resulted in more patients receiving prescriptions on clinic visits and more prescription orders per patient per visit. Also, patients were more likely to have prescriptions dispensed at the pharmacy that required the smallest copayment. Records at four Community Health Association (Michigan) facilities were examined. Since there was felt to be no difference in patient population among the clinics, it was decided to administer questionnaires to eligible and noneligible patients at the nine physician Connor Clinic for one week periods in March, May, September and October 1969.

The drug insurance benefit plan took effect on April 1, 1969 (copayment $2.00, reduced to $1.07 October 1, 1969). Questions included personal and economic data plus information on frequency of clinic visits and number of prescriptions. Eighty per cent of the patients visiting the clinic completed questionnaires. Sixty per cent of the patients were given prescription orders. Relatively more eligible than noneligible patients received prescriptions. Physicians were found to be more likely to prescribe for adult females than adult males, however, after the $1.07 copayment took effect, the physicians increased the number of prescriptions for eligible adult males. In March 1969, 60–70 per cent of the eligible patients had prescriptions dispensed at the clinic pharmacy. After October 1, 1969, when almost any prescription drug could be obtained by eligible patients at the clinic pharmacy for not more than $1.07, more than eighty per cent of the patients received prescriptions. Also, after October 1, 1969, patients received more multiple prescriptions than they did prior to that date. There was a tendency to prescribe more expensive drugs and to increase the size of prescription orders.

References, 0.

WEEKS, H. ASHLEY. *Journal of the American Pharmaceutical Association NS13* (4):205–209, April 1973.

1972

The United Auto Workers Negotiated Prepaid Prescription Drug Program

83

The success of the United Auto Workers (UAW) prepaid prescription drug program, initiated in 1969, has demonstrated the feasibility of a drug prepayment plan on a nationally uniform basis. The plan is primarily administered through a national Blue Cross-Blue Shield arrangement; commercial insurance carriers are used in a few regions of the nation. The Michigan Blue Cross-Blue Shield has responsibility for the administration of the plan. Participating private pharmacists are reimbursed on the basis of "acquisition cost plus a dispensing fee." The basic copayment per prescription is $2. Plan members can patronize a nonparticipating pharmacy, but will generally not be reimbursed 100 per cent (less the $2 copayment). The "problem" areas of the plan and possible future developments offered as solutions to these problems are explored. The three areas needing assessment are: (1) whether a fair price is being paid to the vendor and for the program, (2) whether only drugs which are needed are being prescribed, and (3) whether the program is being administered efficiently. Incentives to the pharmacist to reduce drug costs and the possible establishment of a utilization review and audit control program are discussed.

References, 1, *Key words:* Drug utilization review.

GOLDBERG, THEODORE; and LOREN, EUGENE L. *Journal of the American Pharmaceutical Association NS12* (8):422–425, August 1972.

Effect of Coinsurance: A Multivariate Analysis

179 This study examines the impact of coinsurance upon four variables: physician visits, physician expense, ancillary services and ancillary services expense. The subjects for the study were members of the Palo Alto Group Health Plan. In the study, a 25 per cent coinsurance rate was introduced. It was found that the introduction of this 25 per cent coinsurance reduced physician visits among the subscribers and their dependents by an average of 1.37 visits. Spending for physician services also decreased, but to a lesser degree than the number of physician visits. The data also show that use of ancillary services did not decrease as much as use of physician services. In this study the partial effect of each variable is considered.

References, not counted; footnotes used.

PHELPS, CHARLES E.; and NEWHOUSE, JOSEPH P. *Social Security Bulletin* 35 (6):20–28, 44, June 1972.

Effect of Coinsurance on Use of Physician Services

210 A study of the effects of the imposition of a coinsurance provision on the utilization of physician services in a prepaid medical care plan was conducted at the Group Health Plan in Palo Alto, California. A 25 per cent coinsurance requirement was introduced into the plan in 1967. No other major changes were made in the plan at that time. The study population only included individuals who had been enrolled in the plan for both the entire calendar year prior to the change (1966) and the entire year after the change (1968). Utilization was measured and comparisons were made on a number of dimensions, including socio-economic status, age, sex, type of service utilized, cost of service utilized and place of visit (office or hospital). The specialty of the physicians was also studied.

Results showed that the per capita use of the services of physicians declined 24.1 per cent and the per capita cost declined 23.8 per cent. Hospital-based physician services declined least, while home health visits declined the most. The utilization changes were statistically significant.

The question remains as to whether the coinsurance reduced unnecessary or necessary services. A study of diagnoses indicated that visits for minor conditions declined more than visits for more serious complaints. Also significant was the fact that utilization declined most for the lowest socio-economic group. The authors conclude that, while it is impossible to make a definitive statement, it appears that a 25 per cent coinsurance requirement is too high for the low socio-economic group, since it appears to reduce not only visits for minor complaints, but also the use of services for more serious conditions.

References, 9.

See abstract 209, page 97.

SCITOVSKY, ANNE A.; and SNYDER, NELDA M. *Social Security Bulletin* 35 (6):3–19, June 1972.

Cross-References:

For further information on patient cost sharing, see:

ABSTRACT NUMBER	PAGE NUMBER	ABSTRACT NUMBER	PAGE NUMBER
18	57	141	20
26	54	149	60
27	55	158	8
54	6	160	29
55	6	164	21
56	10	173	49
64	54	176	79
66	56	202	27
73	14	209	97
94	23	212	60
95	106	227	161
97	58	228	162
113	41	244	50
128	167	257	62

VI

Direct Provision of Drugs and Pharmacy Services

The tight controls afforded to a third party by directly providing benefits may produce economies. Examples include programs such as Health Maintenance Organizations operating their own pharmacies or mail-out drug services.
Key words: Direct provision.

1975

Experiences of the New Pharmacy System in Sweden

148

The Swedish pharmacy system since its consolidation under a government-sponsored company is described. A Medicines Act regulates the import, production and quality control of drugs. Pharmacies were regulated private enterprises until 1970, when the Apoteksbolaget AB (National Corporation of Swedish Pharmacies) was created to hold exclusive right to the public distribution of drugs. It bought out all existing pharmacies and their owners became company employees. The company is responsible for ensuring the supply of drugs, disseminating drug research, providing optimal service, charging low and uniform prices that yield a reasonable return, and promoting information and statistics on drugs and drug use. Sweden's 25 counties, which are responsible for health care, cooperate in 7 health care regions. The company has 7 regional offices to service as liaison between its 683 pharmacies (it also has many other drug outlets) and headquarters in Stockholm. Most pharmacies are small; a few very large. Sales were $500 million in 1974.

Staff is about 12,000 in total, 9,700 full-time, and categorized as pharmacists, prescriptionists and technical assistants. To optimize staff productivity, which is up 14 per cent since 1972, doctors of pharmacy are generally chiefs of hospital pharmacies, pharmacists run the biggest community pharmacies, and prescriptionists are in charge of small ones and do most of the dispensing. Ninety-six per cent of prescriptions are delivered immediately; the rest within 24 hours. There has been a 9 per cent increase in the number of pharmacies and 11 per cent have moved to improved locations. Since Apoteksbolaget began wholesaling drugs in 1975, costs for this are probably lower than in any other country. Drug prices have increased, but less than prices in general. The organization's resources have been used to minimize local administrative burdens, e.g., by centralized, computerized payment of wages and invoicing. Apoteksbolaget is testing the use of computer terminals in several pharmacies to prepare labels and record information on prescribing patterns. The company has had a surplus each year except the first. It is just starting on price negotiations with drug companies and expanding efforts at rational drug choice into outpatient care. Contrary to rumors, the system is succeeding. The cooperation of all institutions involved is necessary to attain the best health care.

References, 0.

LÖNNGREN, RUNE. *Journal of the American Pharmaceutical Association NS15* (7):379–381, 405, July 1975.

1974

Inclusion of Pharmaceutical Services in Health Maintenance and Related Organizations: A Review of Supplemental Benefits

95

Health Maintenance Organization (HMO) pharmacy services are discussed in terms of both the medical care system and the internal administration. Supplemental benefits, organizational arrangements for providers of specific services, cost and financing mechanisms, case studies of prototype HMO's (1972–1973)—both group practice and foundation types and other optional services (usually dental and mental health) are all defined. Alternative methods are presented for the inclusion of drug benefits in developing HMO's. (The HMO prototypes analyzed include Group Health Cooperative of Puget Sound (Seattle), Columbia (Maryland) Medical Plan, Metropolitan Health Plan of Detroit, Kaiser Foundation Health Plan of Southern California, Health Insurance Plan of Greater New York, Group Health Association (Washington, D.C.), Detroit Model Neighborhood Comprehensive Health Program, United Mine Workers of America Health and Retirement Funds, San Joaquin (California) Foundation for Medical Care, Group Health Plan of St. Paul (Minnesota).)

Control mechanisms are discussed, such as pharmacy and therapeutics committees, formularies, drug utilization review, patient cost sharing, risk sharing and restrictions on prescribed quantity, and the 1973 American Public Health Association meeting on pharmaceutical services in HMO's is reviewed. In 1970, third-party plans with pharmacy benefits covered 2.12 million persons and paid an estimated $1 billion in benefits, 4 per cent of which was for outpatient prescription drugs. Experience suggests that a minimum population of 4000 enrollees is required to support an HMO-operated pharmacy with one full-time pharmacist.

References, not counted; footnotes used. *Key words:* Drug utilization review, formularies, patient cost sharing

HEALTH SERVICES ADMINISTRATION. DHEW Publication No. (HSA) 74-13017. Washington, D.C., United States Government Printing Office, 1974.

1973

Drug Services and Costs in Health Maintenance Organization Prototypes

111

The accessibility, continuity, quality and efficiency of drug care in 11 privately and publicly funded health maintenance (HMO) programs were studied from December, 1971 to January, 1972 through interviews and published reports. The services analyzed included (1) outpatient provision of prescription drug products (and related factors such as acceptable patient waiting time), (2) prepayment mechanisms, (3) drug utilization review and control (such as the Paid Prescriptions/San Joaquin Foundation system using community pharmacies, as well as additional services such as the maintenance of patient drug profiles), (4) preparation and dissemination of prescription related information beyond required labeling practices, (5) facilitating prescription acquisition (delivery, mail-orders, pharmacy hours of operation), (6) drug education (programs usually limited to "medically indigent" groups, (7) availability of nonprescription drugs and health related products, (8) prescribing by pharmacist when the patient's physician is unavailable.

Of the 11 HMOs studied, only 2 provided formal drug utilization review and control mechanisms; the other 9 indicated that these efforts were undertaken informally. In the area of prepaid prescriptions, all 11 HMOs maintained a formal prepayment mechanism. Paid Prescriptions of San Joaquin uses quantitative prescription utilization data from their prepayment program to establish prescribing and utilization standards. In the area of supplemental drug information, 7 HMOs established formal programs. In general, privately financed systems provided additional information on special prescription labels; public systems serving medically indigent populations provided verbal instructions. The basic drug system made available by HMOs was the provision of the prescription. The most rapidly growing service was the prepaid prescription drug benefit. Drug system costs in the HMOs were analyzed in terms of expenses for facilities, personnel, prescription and nonprescription drug products and equipment, as well as the use of prepaid and copaid drug benefits, pricing methods, number of personnel and prescriptions dispensed. System variation limited comparison, but the data showed that some form of copayment was common. The highest average costs and prescription charges were found in small, decentralized systems. Suggestions were made for research to improve drug system services within HMOs in areas such as drug information, drug distribution, decision-making activities of health care providers and organizations, and patient behavior.

References, 24. *Key words:* Drug utilization review

JOHNSON, RICHARD E.; and CAMPBELL, WILLIAM H. *American Journal of Hospital Pharmacy 30* (5):405–421, May 1973.

The Mail-Order Prescription Drug Industry

255

Six general features of the services of the mail-order prescription drug industry are discussed: patient characteristics, prescription pricing, prescription processing, prescription dispensing, prescription shipping and prescription volume and drugs dispensed. The industry profile was compiled from a survey of ten of the largest mail-order prescription suppliers. These ten organizations, selected from a listing of the sixty known mail-order suppliers, are responsible for about 90 per cent of the total volume of mail-order prescription drugs in the United States (estimated at 17 million prescriptions annually).

A standard set of questions was used in the survey, which was conducted through personal and telephone interviews. A few of the many specific characteristics of the services discussed were: (1) most mail-order suppliers serve elderly patients with chronic conditions, who use many drugs, and who live in rural areas, (2) mail-order prices are generally competitive with drug prices in urban areas: some organizations offer a discount on prescription prices to their members, (3) firms generally take precautionary steps to screen out fraudulent orders, (4) most organizations do not maintain drug-use profiles of patients, nor perform drug interaction monitoring of their patient's drug regimens and (5) drug dispensing operations are supervised by pharmacists.

Specific services offered by individual suppliers are discussed. For example, the Veterans Administration program is unique in that it is the only organization allowed by postal regulations to dispense narcotics through the mails. A discussion follows on two issues which are generally raised by opponents of the mail-order industry: the alleged disruption of the traditional physician-patient-pharmacist relationship, and the potential for fraud in prescription mail-orders. There is a lack of factual evidence to support or disprove these claims. The authors suggest that the economic competition of the mail-order suppliers may force retail pharmacists to oppose them. An objective evaluation of practices and the development of standards for the prescription mail-order industry is recommended.

References, 6.

WERTHEIMER, ALBERT, I.; and KNOBEN, JAMES E. *Health Services Reports 88* (9):852–856, November 1973.

1972

Pharmacy Involvement in the Neighborhood Health Center Environment

184 The planning, development and implementation of a neighborhood health center pharmacy service in Tucson, Arizona is described in detail. The service was developed by the University of Arizona College of Pharmacy. The health center is located in a low-income area predominantly populated by Mexican-Americans. The administration of the health center is discussed. Planning for the pharmacy program was done in close cooperation with representatives of the community and with community pharmacists. The program involves a combination system of in-house and vendor pharmacy services. The in-house facility provides a full range of pharmaceutical services and maintains a patient data record for all medications prescribed and dispensed for each patient, regardless of whether the drug is obtained at the in-house Center pharmacy or at a vendor pharmacy. Guidelines for vendor pharmacies provide control over the quality and quantity of services offered, the cost of prescriptions, the items contained in the vendor's formulary and prescription renewal procedures.

Thirty-six of the seventy-six community pharmacies in Tucson are vendor pharmacies. A Grievance Committee has been established to ensure good communication between the neighborhood health center pharmacy and the vendor pharmacies. All parties benefit educationally from the program: vendor pharmacists are required to attend programs instituted by the Center, and students in the College of Pharmacy have the opportunity to obtain on-the-job experience while receiving college credit.

References, 6.

ROBLES, RAMON R.; and WINSHIP, HENRY W. III. *American Journal of Hospital Pharmacy* 29 (1):68–71, January 1972.

1971

Pharmacy and the Poor

1

This is a report on the first 2 years of a project funded by the Office of Economic Opportunity on pharmacy services for neighborhood health centers. Residents of poverty areas and the pharmacies available to them were surveyed in five urban locations and one rural location. Few differences were found between poor and nonpoor residents and between poverty area and nonpoverty area pharmacies in terms of size and number of prescriptions dispensed, age of pharmacist, prices charged for selected prescriptions and services requested from the pharmacist. The pharmacist was not viewed as a person to consult for advice on health matters.

Pharmacy systems examined included health centers with on-site pharmacies staffed by more than one pharmacist using the team approach to health care, health centers with on-site pharmacies staffed by more than two pharmacists and having a high daily prescription volume, health centers which purchased pharmaceutical services from community pharmacies, and prepaid group medical practices with their own pharmacies. An on-site pharmacy does not always mean greater services for patients or prescribers, greater convenience for patients, an expanded role for the pharmacist, or an adverse economic impact on area pharmacies. An on-site pharmacy does mean low cost to the health center per prescription, greater opportunity for control and greater educational and professional potential for the pharmacist. An off-site pharmacy means greater cost, more effort required for program controls, and a favorable economic impact on contractors.

References, 44.

AMERICAN PHARMACEUTICAL ASSOCIATION. Washington, D.C., The Association, 1971.

The Prepaid Group Practice Point of View

29

The Health Insurance Plan (HIP) of New York, a nonprofit comprehensive health care package, is modelled on already existing prepaid group practice plans which facilitate the rational prescribing and dispensing of drugs. In addition to paying, HIP arranges the availability, suitability and quality of care, and serves 780,000 persons in and around New York through 30 physician partnerships under contract to HIP. Extensive services are offered and, as drugs are purchased in bulk, costs are lower and quality is carefully monitored. An HIP-operated mail-order service has, since 1968, offered the highest quality drugs. Through bulk purchase, drugs are obtained at a saving that independent pharmacies cannot match. HIP has the only licensed pharmacy which has a drug control board that makes recommendations on matters concerning dispensing, improving quality control, etc. At present they are working on creating a drug formulary and they will soon implement a computerized system which will provide both operational and research data and will aid in compiling a medical profile for every HIP patient. Experience has shown that linking drug programs to medical care provided by health personnel allows for the alleviation of problems relating to the dispensing of drugs at low cost with appropriate quality control. This will only be realized when there is sufficient coordination among the many organizational units.

References, 0. *Key words:* Formularies.

BRINDLE, JAMES; and WOLMAN, MILTON H. *Journal of the American Pharmaceutical Association NS11* (2):68–70, February 1971.

1968

Prepayment of Drug Costs under a Group Practice Prepayment Plan

154 The outpatient prescription drug program described is a part of the comprehensive prepaid health plan of the Group Health Cooperative of Puget Sound in Seattle, Washington. Three characteristics of the drug program which help reduce drug costs are: (1) the development and adherence to a drug formulary, (2) the control of drug use by the Pharmacy Committee and central administration and (3) economies permitted due to the size of the program, e.g., the bulk lot purchase of drugs by generic name. The specific features of the drug formulary are discussed. One important aspect of it is the inclusion of cost estimates for particular amounts of each drug which are found alongside the drug product listing in the formulary and which enable the physician to compare costs vs. benefits when prescribing. The organization of the pharmacy committee and its responsibilities in the evaluation of proposed and current formulary products is discussed. The nature of the group practice enables the drug prescription practices of all members to be monitored and ensures that each physician knows all the drugs currently prescribed for each patient.

The economic aspects of the pharmacies' operations (there are four pharmacies in the organization) are discussed in detail. Drug purchases are made in large volumes and by generic name whenever possible. Some drugs and medications are manufactured in the pharmacies. Costs are reduced by job specialization and the employment of pharmacy clerks. Extensive data on pharmacy costs (1966) are presented. In 1966, the average annual per capita cost for prescription drugs for the cooperative's members was $8.80, which was 45 per cent less than the average annual per capita cost of prescription drugs in the United States. Factors which could account for such a significant difference are: (1) the nonprofit and tax-exempt nature of the cooperative, (2) the data assume that a member's prescription drugs are all acquired at a pharmacy of the cooperative, (3) lack of delivery and credit services offered by the pharmacy, the availability of which increases prescription drug costs in retail pharmacies, (4) economies due to size of operation, and (5) control over drug prescribing and utilization. With adjustments made for differences in the operation, coverage and services between the prepaid drug program and the retail pharmacy, the per capita cost for prescription drugs for cooperative members is estimated to be 25 per cent–30 per cent less than the average annual per capita cost of prescription drugs in the United States.

References, 9. *Key words:* Drug utilization review, formularies.

McCAFFREE, KENNETH M.; and NEWMAN, HAROLD F. *American Journal of Public Health* 58 (7):1212–1218, July 1968.

1966

Impact of a Reduced Charge Drug Benefit in a Prepaid Group Practice Plan

88

A reduced charge out-of-hospital drug benefit made available in October 1962 to the 83,000 members of the Oregon region of the Kaiser Foundation Health Plan resulted in an increase in the use of plan pharmacies and lower drug costs to members. This prepaid group practice includes subscribers from diverse socioeconomic and occupational groups, and provides a full range of services at a hospital clinic and two neighborhood clinics, each with its own pharmacy. The clinic, a partnership of more than 60 full-time specialists, receives a fee per capita per month from the health plan. The plan pharmacies, under a prescription price discounting program, earned 18 per cent per member per month, and it was decided to reduce this revenue to the break even point. The clinic agreed to reduce capitation fees so that the drug benefit could be offered to members at no additional cost, and with minimal loss of revenue to the plan. Prices were set at *Blue Book* cost plus 60¢ on October 1, 1962, and reduced to *Blue Book* cost plus 30¢ on June 1 1963, with a minimum price of $1.25. Prescriptions dispensed per physician visit for the hospital clinic from 1960–1964 show a downward trend before the benefit was implemented and an upward trend thereafter. This is not attributed to a change in prescribing habits but to the increased utilization of the plan pharmacies because of their lower prices (a 39.1 per cent increase in number of dispensed prescriptions per member per year). Data show average savings to members of 31.3 per cent per prescription for 1964. Net income per member month from the pharmacy was reduced by 50.1 per cent but still returned revenue to the plan.

References, 0. *Key words:* Reimbursement.

GREENLICK, MERWYN R.; and SAWARD, ERNEST W. *Public Health Reports 81* (10):938–940, October 1966.

Cross-References

For further information on direct provision of services, see:

ABSTRACT NUMBER	PAGE NUMBER	ABSTRACT NUMBER	PAGE NUMBER
16	34	170	160
37	65	181	162
87	81	256	178

VII

Drug Cost Controls: Maximum Allowable Cost Program

The Maximum Allowable Cost (MAC) program is the first major federal initiative to reduce drug product cost in government programs. It establishes MACs for multi-source products, Estimated Acquisition Costs for all other drugs, and provides for drug cost information to be distributed to prescribers.
Key words: Maximum allowable cost.

1977

Limits on Drug Reimbursements To Save Millions

11

This article presents, in interview format, a discussion of the Maximum Allowable Cost (MAC) regulations by three federal officials concerned with the program. They are Vincent Gardner, Chief of the Drug Studies Branch of the Health Care Financing Administration, Mark Novitch, Deputy Associate Commissioner for Medical Affairs for the Food and Drug Administration and Henry Spiegelblatt, Director of the Division of Policy and Standards of the Health Care Financing Administration.

The conversation addresses many points related to the Maximum Allowable Cost program in easy to understand terms. Some of the points discussed include: the number of drugs to be included in the MAC program (around 50); the process of establishing a MAC for a particular product; the time necessary to establish one MAC (3 to 5 months); methods for revising MAC prices; court cases involving the MAC regulations; the composition of the MAC Advisory Committee and the internal MAC Board; methods of establishing pharmacist dispensing fees; the role of the states in implementing the program; the education which physicians receive related to brand and generic drugs; and the proposed price guide for physicians and pharmacists.

References, 0.

ANONYMOUS. *Record 1* (3):13–17, June 1977.

The Maximum Allowable Cost Program and Wholesale Drug Prices, a Preliminary Analysis

52

Beginning in 1974, drug prices rose significantly (with the percentage increase greater for single source than multiple source drugs) largely because of (1) price increases for petroleum based chemicals and other drug components resulting, in part, from the 1973 oil embargo, and (2) the lifting of federal price controls in 1973, which allowed drug manufacturers to increase prices more sharply than had been the case in the previous few years. It is also suggested that manufacturers of single source drugs took advantage of their economic position and thus raised prices to increase their revenues; economic competition for multiple source drugs prevented price increases of similar magnitude for these products.

It has been alleged that the rapid rise in drug prices since 1974 was a reaction by drug manufacturers to HEW's Maximum Allowable Cost (MAC) program (announced in July 1975), which established its first price ceiling (on ampicillin capsules) in June 1977. Analysis of Consumer Price Index (CPI) data for prescriptions and Wholesale Price Index (WPI) data for pharmaceuticals for 1970–1976 (first half) indicates that the most significant price increases occurred in 1974, too soon to be explained as a reaction to proposed MAC regulations. Wholesale price data for the 300 most frequently prescribed single source drugs and the 300 most frequently prescribed multiple source drugs for the first quarter of 1976 were extracted. A sample of 65 brand name products was selected from these and the annual price changes computed for 1970–1976 (first half). The CPI/WPI data and the wholesale price change data for a sample of drugs both fail to support the suggestion that the MAC program caused price increases. Had this been the case, the sharpest increases would have appeared in late 1975 rather than 1974, as was shown.

References, 1.

DICKENS, PAUL F.; and HOGAN, TIMOTHY D. Research and Statistics. Note No. 11. Washington, D.C., Social Security Administration, July 12, 1977.

Drug Cost Control: The Road to the Maximum Allowable Cost Regulations

73

The more than 15 years of Congressional investigation of the pharmaceutical industry and the increasing involvement of the federal government in financing health care programs is reviewed as background to the development of the Maximum Allowable Cost (MAC) regulations on drug costs. The Kefauver hearings (1959–62), the Nelson hearings (1967–), the HEW Task Force on Prescription Drugs (1967–69) and the Kennedy hearings (1973–), all focused attention on the lack of price competition for pharmaceuticals fostered by the 17-year period of patent protection for new drugs. However, growing interest in generic prescribing is encouraging price competition for multisource drugs. This has led to a controversy over the chemical and therapeutic equivalence of drug products and standards for drug quality, and to criticism of the consistently high profits in the pharmaceutical industry, notwithstanding legitimate research and development expenditures. Legislation in 1962 required proof of efficacy for new drug products and 1972 legislation limited physician and hospital charges and established Professional Standards Review Organizations for Medicare/Medicaid programs.

Two approaches to drug cost control have been considered: (1) utilization review, and (2) more cost effective reimbursement programs. Utilization review studies reveal problems such as inappropriate prescribing and adverse drug reactions. Cost effectiveness studies focus on copayment programs. Thus, the need to improve cost effectiveness in Medicare/Medicaid programs led to the development of the MAC regulations, including mechanisms for reviewing bioequivalence through the FDA and for setting price limits on multisource drugs through the Pharmaceutical Reimbursement Board and the Pharmaceutical Reimbursement Advisory Committee. In addition, HEW will provide information on the costs of frequently prescribed drugs to assist states in estimating the actual cost to the pharmacist of prescription drugs, rather than retail cost, for use as the basis for reimbursement. The success of such procedures for drug cost containment is seen as having considerable impact on the future of national health insurance legislation.

References, 34. *Key words:* Drug utilization review, patient cost sharing.

FULDA, THOMAS R. *In* Friedman, Kenneth; and Rakoff, Stuart. *Toward a National Health Policy, Public Policy in the Control of Health Care Costs.* Lexington, Massachusetts, Lexington Books, 1977. Pages 55–67.

Policy Implications of Maximum Allowable Cost: Average Wholesale Price and Actual Acquisition Cost Differentials Among Pharmacies

168

The drug product costs of a representative sample of 100 Iowa pharmacies were studied from December 1975 to April 1976. The mean differential between average wholesale price (AWP) and actual acquisition cost (AAC) was $0.56 per prescription (17.5 per cent of the mean AAC per prescription). A reimbursement schedule based on AAC would thus represent considerable savings to HEW and state Medicaid programs.

Analysis of the data by various pharmacy characteristics indicated that: (1) chain pharmacies have mean AWP-AAC differentials of $0.70, a result of their large volume orders, (2) promotional discount pharmacies have mean AWP-AAC differentials of $0.72, which may be a function of ownership as well as prescription volume and (3) high prescription volume pharmacies (over 30,000 prescriptions per year) have mean AWP-AAC differentials of $0.65, as opposed to the AWP-AAC differential of very low volume pharmacies (less than 10,000 prescriptions per year) of $0.42.

A system which establishes a standardized price for reimbursement would discriminate against those pharmacies unable to purchase products in large quantities. A system based on AAC or an adjusted estimated acquisition cost (EAC) would eliminate this purchasing advantage.

References, 5.

NORWOOD, G. JOSEPH; LIPSON, DAVID P.; and FREEMAN, ROBERT A. *Journal of the American Pharmaceutical Association NS17* (8):496–499, August 1977.

1976

The Maximum Allowable Cost Regulations and Pharmaceutical Research and Development

51

The Maximum Allowable Cost (MAC) regulations, effective July 25, 1975, provide that Medicare, Medicaid and other HEW programs will reimburse for multisource drug products at or below the price established by the Pharmaceutical Reimbursement Board of HEW. This price will be the lowest at which a particular drug product is widely and consistently available. Annual savings from this program are estimated at $37.2 million. The immediate effect of MAC will be to channel government funds into lower priced products. Also, reimbursement to pharmacies will be based on an estimate of actual price paid (plus dispensing fee) rather than on list price (the latter found to be 15–18 per cent higher than the actual price paid); this action is expected to save $23.1–$38.4 million annually. HEW will publish a price list for frequently prescribed drugs by therapeutic category. This information (modeled on the Ontario, Canada PARCOST program) is expected to encourage cost consciousness in prescribing and dispensing.

The effect of these actions on pharmaceutical research and development (R&D) is demonstrated in three models of the pharmaceutical industry. In the "industrialist" model, where the research and development is funded from current profits, the MAC regulations are expected to reduce R&D expenditures as profits on existing drug products decline. In the model in which R&D is financed through capital expenditures rather than current earnings, the potential negative effects of MAC are minimized. In the "managerial" model, the MAC program may encourage R&D. The optimal level of R&D expenditures in this model is assumed to be that which will produce a sufficient number of new drug products to maintain a predetermined corporate rate of return satisfactory to management and investors. Since MAC may reduce the current rate of return, management may desire to increase investment in R&D in an attempt to restore the optimal level, since R&D expenditures are expected to yield higher priced patent-protected products.

References, 6.

DICKENS, PAUL F. III. Research and Statistics Note No. 2-1976. Office of Research and Statistics. Social Security Administration. DHEW Pub. No. (SSA) 76-11701. Washington, D.C., United States Government Printing Office, March 4, 1976.

Maximum Allowable Cost and Estimated Acquisition Cost—The View from Washington

79

The unexpectedly large impact of Medicare and Medicaid on health care costs has created concern about federal drug reimbursement programs. Between 1967 and 1975, drug reimbursements under Medicare rose from $241 million to $1.1 billion and federal Medicaid drug payments from $186 million to $877 million. The government must both shift more costs to recipients and achieve greater cost effectiveness.

The three-part Maximum Allowable Cost (MAC) program will help reduce costs. The first part involves determining the maximum practical reimbursement levels for selected multiple source drug products. The second limits drug reimbursements to state estimates of pharmacist acquisiton cost plus an appropriate dispensing fee. States may use either actual acquisition costs (AAC) or an estimated acquisition cost (EAC) based on the price generally paid for the most frequently purchased package size in that state. The Federal Government is supplying the results of a national survey of invoice costs for the most common drugs solely for guidance.

The February price list was not current enough but it will help states set up their programs. The Federal Government is working on a second update and will continue publishing monthly price data. Although 60 per cent of its prices are at *Red Book* average wholesale price, the EAC program is warranted by wide disparity in pharmacists' costs. Preliminary guidelines for state surveys of pharmacy operating costs went out in March. The Federal Government realizes some states are reluctant to adjust pharmacy dispensing fees, but HEW cannot recommend mandated fee levels without much more data. It is grossly unfair that drug price increases pass through the Medicaid program while pharmacist fees are limited because of fiscal constraints. The author requests help in finding a solution. The third part of the MAC program just calls for twice-a-year publication of drug product price information for physicians and pharmacists. Though the author looks ultimately to peer review and pharmacy consultants to improve care and reduce expenditures, success with current cost control efforts is politically prerequisite to any new programs. The MAC regulations recognize the unique role of pharmaceutical services. Pharmacists can justify more equitable payment levels by contributing as part of the health care team to more rational and cost effective therapy.

References, 0.

GARDNER, VINCE. *California Pharmacist* 24 (*1*):36–39, July 1976.

1975

Evolution of the Final Maximum Allowable Cost Regulations

7

On January 16, 1974, the American Pharmaceutical Association (APhA) endorsed the general concept of the new federal reimbursement policy. Between then and November 15, 1974, when the first specific regulations were published in the *Federal Register*, the Office of Technology Assessment studied the complex area of bioavailability. APhA's response to the report was cited in the APhA journal. Further regulations were published several times through February 15, 1975. At its annual meeting in San Francisco in April 1975, the APhA House of Delegates voted approval of the Association's formal response. Final Maximum Allowable Cost regulations were issued by the resigning Secretary of HEW, Caspar Weinberger, on July 28, 1975. While the regulations became effective July 31, 1975, Section 19.3 dealing with cost limitations became effective April 26, 1976 (later deferred again).

References, 0.

ANONYMOUS. *Journal of the American Pharmaceutical Association* NS15 (*9*):506–526, September 1975.

Maximum Allowable Cost Program— A Close-up Look

252 HEW Secretary Caspar Weinberger appeared before the American Pharmaceutical Association in April 1975 to discuss the Maximum Allowable Cost (MAC) program. He reported that over 2,600 comments regarding the regulations had been received since they were published, which indicates that the regulations are highly controversial.

He pointed out, however, that the federal government spends over $2.5 billion per year on procuring drug products, and thus has a justifiable interest in holding costs down. HEW estimates that it can save $89 million dollars a year under the MAC program. Even more will be saved if a drug benefit under a national health insurance program is adopted.

In constructing the MAC regulations, HEW recognized that physicians lack drug price comparison data, so they cannot choose the best drug at the lowest available price. The MAC program will make available a list of estimated acquisition costs for all drugs, along with limitation of reimbursement for multisource products to the lowest price of those generally available. Finally, comparative pricing information will be made available to practicing physicians and pharmacists.

Suitable safeguards are built into the program. Physicians who wish their patients to receive a specified drug may so indicate. All drugs will be reviewed for bioequivalence problems by the Food and Drug Administration before MAC limits are proposed. The MAC regulations will not overrule state laws related to substitution. The regulations are seen by HEW as the best approach to controlling drug costs while tampering as little as possible with the free enterprise system.

References, 0.

WEINBERGER, CASPAR W. *Journal of the American Pharmaceutical Association NS 15* (7):376–377, July 1975.

Cross-References

For further information on Maximum Allowable Cost, see:

VIII

Drug Cost Controls: Product Selection and Substitution among Multisource Products

---

Many states have repealed or modified laws which prohibited pharmacists from selecting a supplier for multiple source drugs if prescribed by brand name. Product selection by pharmacists, adding economic criteria to therapeutic ones, could help to contain the cost of drug products.
Key word: Substitution.

1977

Impact of Drug Substitution Legislation: A Report of the First Year's Experience

82

Analysis of data collected after the passage of a "generically equivalent" drug substitution law in Michigan showed four main findings: (1) more than 50 per cent of all prescription orders written were for multiple source drug products, thus allowing ample opportunity for generic substitution, (2) 18.9 per cent of multiple source drug prescriptions were written generically; generic substitution for these prescriptions was permitted before passage of the new law, (3) only 6.4 per cent of prescriptions required that they be dispensed only as written, and (4) actual substitution of a generically equivalent product occurred for less than 0.75 per cent of all prescription orders and for only 1.5 per cent of all prescriptions for multiple source drugs.

Data were collected from random samples of prescriptions dispensed at community pharmacies in Michigan and Wisconsin. Pharmacies with different characteristics (e.g., geographic location) were surveyed. A second sample for year two of the study consisted of the ten prescription records following each randomly selected prescription; data were recorded from these ten prescriptions only if a substitution was made. The data were analyzed according to frequency distribution of prescriptions by generic category and by drug entity.

The very low percentage of actual generic substitution may be a result of poor communication between the pharmacist and the patient.

References, 2.

GOLDBERG, THEODORE; ALDRIDGE, GERALD W.; DeVITO, CAROLEE A.; VIDIS, JERRY; MOORE, WILLIS E.; and DICKSON, W. MICHAEL. *Journal of the American Pharmaceutical Association NS17* (4):216–226, April 1977.

Relationship of Price to Bioavailability for Four Multiple Source Drug Products

221 The study found little correlation between the cost and bioavailability of four generic drug products: nitrofurantoin (50 mg and 100 mg), propoxyphenes and tetracyclines. The correlation coefficients were 0.01 (nitrofurantoins), 0.40 (tetracyclines) and 0.62 (propoxyphenes). The pharmacist cannot rely on price as an indicator of drug product quality. There was only one case (two 50 mg nitrofurantoin products) in which significant bioavailability differences were found among generic products.

References, 8. *Key words:* Maximum allowable cost.

SLYWKA, GERALD W.A.; RYAN, MICHAEL R.; MELIKIAN, ARMEN P.; MEYER, MARVIN C.; BATES, HERBERT E.; and WHYATT, PHILIP L. *Journal of the American Pharmaceutical Association NS17* (1):30–32, January 1977.

1976

Holders of Approved New Drug Applications for Drugs Presenting Actual or Potential Bioequivalence Problems

67 Holders of approved New Drug Applications (NDAs) or Abbreviated New Drug Applications (ANDAs) for drug products that may have bioequivalency problems are listed in an alphabetical arrangement by generic drug name. These drug manufacturers and distributors have met federal legal requirements for marketing the drug and have submitted bioavailability data where possible. The FDA suggests that, until final bioequivalency regulations on these products are determined, drugs be selected by physicians, pharmacists and state health care agencies only from the firms listed. Information on dosage form and strength is included.

References, 0. *Key words:* Maximum allowable cost.

FOOD AND DRUG ADMINISTRATION. HEW Publication No. (FDA) 76-3009. Rockville, Maryland, Food and Drug Administration, June 1976.

Evaluation of Impact of Drug Substitution Legislation

84 Wayne State University's college of medicine and faculty of pharmacy have undertaken a four-year study to analyze prescriptions dispensed in Michigan, a state with relatively lenient drug substitution legislation, and in a similar state not permitting substitution in order to determine the effects of legislation enacted to reduce drug costs through the substitution of cheaper generically equivalent drugs for prescribed brand name drugs. This is a report on some findings of a preliminary survey of related attitudes of Michigan physicians and pharmacists suggesting possible substantial barriers to the effectiveness of the current law. Professional attitudes are significant because, although Michigan's law sets no limits on which generically equivalent lower cost drugs may or may not be substituted, it does require that the physician not preclude substitution and that the pharmacist choose to substitute. (Also, the consumer must request substitution and must realize the savings if the purchase is not covered by a third-party contract.)

Physicians and pharmacists licensed to practice in Michigan in Fall 1974 were divided into 4 regional groups representing Blue Shield's economic divisions of the state and random samples were chosen from each group. Responses to mailed questionnaires were received from 812 (71.2 per cent) of the physicians and 665 (79.7 per cent) of the pharmacists. Usable returns were 646 and 533 respectively. Physicians are 34 per cent pro the legislation and 44.5 per cent con; pharmacists, 50 per cent pro and 38.2 per cent con. About half of each group thinks generic equivalency is essentially the same as therapeutic equivalency for all but a few products. On the key presumption that pharmacists possess the technical knowledge to substitute safely, 82.5 per cent of the pharmacists and 60 per cent of the physicians agree. The same percentage of physicians say their decision on whether to permit substitution will be influenced, at least in part, by a knowledge of the pharmacist involved. Almost 56 per cent of the physicians will encourage selective or general substitutions; almost 9 per cent will actively discourage it. Most physicians, either sometimes or often, prescribe generically now, so potential savings may be less than anticipated. The average correct identification of generic equivalents of a list of 7 drugs was about 57 per cent for pharmacists and less than 30 per cent for physicians. This finding requires further analysis.

Physician responses to another interesting set of questions concerning the prices of commonly prescribed drugs are not yet analyzed, but suggest a wide range in accuracy. An illustrative analysis of the question about whether physicians intend to limit substitution indicates, for example, a correlation between restrictiveness and doctors of osteopathy, general practitioners, frequent prescribers, and those confident of their knowledge of drug prices.

References, 0.

GOLDBERG, THEODORE; MOORE, WILLIS E.; KOONTZ, THEODORE; FACIONE, FRANK; ALDRIDGE, GERALD; VIDIS, JERRY; VADASY, PATRICIA; and JONES, GAIL. *Journal of the American Pharmaceutical Association NS16* (2):64–70, 90, February 1976.

Innovation in the Pharmaceutical Industry

208

An economic analysis of the drug industry is presented, especially the costs of pharmaceutical research. Empirical evidence is examined and recommendations are offered. The book contains chapters on methodology, basic research and invention, characteristics of drug research, importance of industrial sources of new drugs, research activity and the size of the firm, competition by innovation, expected rate of return on pharmaceutical research and development, life of drug patents, promotional expenditures, quality of drugs and generic prescribing, price competition, the economic literature, and government and alternative goals for public policy. It reports that a large proportion of prescriptions for multisource drugs are generic; since pharmacists can and do dispense multisource prescriptions with low-priced drugs (whether written for brand or generic name), price competition is encouraged. Such substitution is surprisingly large, even though illegal in most states. The effectiveness of the FDA and the National Center for Drug Analysis is evaluated. Maximum Allowable Cost regulations, expected to reduce the cost of drugs to the government, plus proposed legislation on formularies, generic drugs and patent rights are discussed. An appendix deals briefly with controversies on drug choice in hypertension, schizophrenia and diabetes.

Key words: Formularies, maximum allowable cost, patents and prices.

SCHWARTZMAN, DAVID. Baltimore, Johns Hopkins University Press, 1976.

The Substitution Controversy: Attitudes of Pharmacists Toward Repeal of Antisubstitution Laws

211 To describe and predict pharmacists' attitudes toward antisubstitution laws and their repeal, a 40-item "Attitude Toward Antisubstitution Laws Scale" (A Scale) was included in a questionnaire mailed nationally to 5000 pharmacists; the response rate was 17 per cent. The data were subjected to considerable statistical treatment.

The A Scale items were developed from the professional literature on the antisubstitution controversy and were summarized by eight factors: competence for brand selection; physician autonomy/derivation of pharmacist prerogatives; therapeutic equivalency; economics of brand selection control; ethics of brand selection; identification and professional regulation of brand selection abusers; pharmacist autonomy/essential pharmacist services; role of the professional organization. The data support the contention that the issue of pharmacist autonomy, more than any possible economic consequences, affects pharmacists' attitudes toward antisubstitution repeal. Repeal of the antisubstitution laws was favored by 72 per cent (610) of the respondents.

References, 15.

SHARPE, THOMAS R.; and SMITH, MICKEY C. *Drugs in Health Care* 3 (*1*):19–34, Winter 1976.

The Massachusetts Drug Formulary Act

245 The provisions of the 1970 Massachusetts Drug Formulary Act, if applied by pharmacies to support generic prescribing and a bid system for the purchase of drug products, will result in savings for pharmacists and consumers, as well as improved inventory control. The Act (included as Appendix A of this paper) requires physicians to include generic or chemical names when prescribing drugs by brand name and creates a commission to develop a formulary of therapeutically equivalent generic substitutes for commonly prescribed brand name drugs. Before the Act was passed, pharmacists were required to dispense the drug product specified. With generic prescribing, however, the pharmacist can dispense equivalent drugs from any manufacturer. If a prescription does not specify the generic name as well as the brand name, pharmacists must contact the physician and request it.

Limitations of the Act are (1) the formulary covers only a limited number of drug products, so pharmacists cannot dispense chemically equivalent drugs that are not listed, (2) physicians may indicate "no substitute" or "brand only" and thus not allow the pharmacist to substitute drug products, (3) there is no enforcement or penalty provision for physicians who do not include generic names when prescribing by brand name and pharmacists will not always contact physicians to obtain this information.

Compliance in 1972 was estimated at greater than 10 per cent. If pharmacists actively employed the guidelines of the Act, they could reduce inventory and costs. Since pharmacists have the authority to substitute equivalent drug products under generic prescribing, they do not have to maintain inventories of several brands of a product. By requesting bids from manufacturers, selecting the best brand (in terms of equivalency and price) and purchasing that brand in a greater quantity, the pharmacy can guarantee a certain market for the manufacturer (perhaps allowing for reduced manufacturing costs) and obtain the product at a reduced unit cost. A sample form for requesting bids is provided. Thus, if the guidelines of the Act are followed, savings on drug costs will result.

References, 5.

TAUBMAN, ALBERT H.; and GOSSELIN, RAYMOND A. *Journal of the American Pharmaceutical Association NS16* (2):71–73, February 1976.

1975

How to Pay Less for Prescription Drugs

9

Despite assurance of therapeutic as well as chemical equivalence, physicians prefer to prescribe brand name rather than generic drugs. Studies show that sales of relatively expensive brand name products account for considerably more of the market than inexpensive generic drugs, even when both agents may be manufactured by the same company. The Pharmaceutical Manufacturers Association (PMA) disagrees with the HEW position on measuring therapeutic equivalence of prescription drugs by determining bioavailability (the amount of active ingredient absorbed in the bloodstream). Drug manufacturers also argue that high prices are necessary to cover research and development costs and that the high risk of scientific research justifies high profits.

HEW questions the risk claimed and notes that drug firms are relatively stable and have exhibited a steady growth in earnings over the years. In addition, HEW calls much drug industry research a "waste" of manpower and facilities; an FDA study of more than 800 drugs introduced between 1950 and 1973 shows that two-thirds of these products offer little or no therapeutic advantage over existing products. The 17-year period of exclusive patent protection rewards drug manufacturers with high prices and brand name identifiability which long outlasts the patent period. The drug industry spends $5000 per private practitioner to promote brand name prescribing, thus enabling drug manufacturers to influence prescribing habits and maintain high drug prices. Antisubstitution laws, now being challenged in the United States Congress, also support brand name prescribing and high drug prices.

The Canadian approach to drug pricing is cited; this includes product selection laws, under which pharmacists may substitute lower priced generic or brand name equivalents for prescribing drugs, and a Comparable Drug Index—a list of approved interchangeable drugs and their prices. To cut prescription costs, consumers should ask physicians to prescribe by generic name and to prescribe drugs for chronic conditions in large quantity, and should compare prices in several pharmacies before having a prescription filled.

References, 0. *Key words:* Other countries.

ANONYMOUS. *Consumer Reports 40* (*1*):48–53, January 1975.

12

Many Oppose Substitution, Survey Shows

A G.D. Searle nationwide survey found that 67 per cent of the people polled were opposed to allowing pharmacists to substitute alternative drugs for the ones prescribed; 29 per cent were in favor and 4 per cent had no opinion. When the alternative drug was less expensive, the number opposed rose to 71 per cent and approval dropped to 25 per cent. Seventy-five per cent of lower-class and poverty-level households, but only 59 per cent of the most affluent, opposed allowing cheaper substitutions. In questions relevant to HEW's proposed maximum allowable cost plan, surveyors first established that 88 per cent of the respondents definitely favored government payment for drugs for the poor and/or elderly. When asked whether the government should pay for any brand of drug prescribed or only for those brands with prices under a certain limit, 68 per cent opted for paying for prescribed brands, 27 per cent favored price limits and 5 per cent had no opinion. The percentage favoring payment for any brand was 60 in affluent households, 73 in poverty-level households and 68 in households without employed workers.

A similar Eli Lilly survey in Wisconsin found that 78 per cent think the physician should determine what drug product is to be used and only 12 per cent favor pharmacist choice. Sixty-four per cent were for retaining antisubstitution laws and 23 per cent opposed them. Others gave qualified answers or no opinion. Only 15 per cent would allow pharmacist substitution, while 76 per cent wanted the drug prescribed. If told the alternative was cheaper, those who would oppose substitution remained the same, but the number who would permit substitution rose to 20 per cent. This increase came from those who had previously given qualified answers. As to who should authorize substitution, 77 per cent held out for the physician, 3 per cent said the pharmacist should be able to decide on his own, and 15 per cent would personally accept a switch if the pharmacist discussed the reason for it. When asked for the most important aspect of prescription drugs, 56 per cent said safety of use; 42 per cent, quality and/or effectiveness; and only 4 per cent, cost.

References, 0. *Key words:* Maximum allowable cost.

ANONYMOUS. *Drug Topics 119* (*12*):6, June 16, 1975.

Resistant Prices: A Study of Competitive Strains in the Antibiotic Markets

34

The prices paid by drug stores for multisource antibiotics from 8 major firms are examined. The book contains chapters on prices and the provision of drugs (especially antibiotics), bioequivalence, methods of analysis, the antibiotic markets, drug store prices, and firm prices and premiums. The author considers Maximum Allowable Cost the only current mechanism for reporting and controlling drug store prices charged to consumers; these prices reflect how suppliers control the drug market. Published prices, drug store prices and hospital prices are discussed and it was noted that antisubstitution laws require pharmacies to stock the best known (and therefore more expensive) products, resulting in less demand for less expensive products. It is suggested that generic prescribing involves price, not quality, factors relating to patent protection and competition. Appendices on sources, the wholesale adjustment factor, and firm, drug store and hospital sales (1973) are included.

References, not counted; footnotes used. *Key words:* Maximum allowable cost, patents and prices.

BROOKE, PAUL A. New York, Council on Economic Priorities, 1975.

New Professional Liability Problems? Legal Implications of Generic Drug Substitution

42

Dr. Chewning presents four arguments against the practice of generic drug substitution by the pharmacist: (1) difficulty in the assignment of legal liability should an adverse reaction to the drug product occur, (2) lack of federal standards or regulatory programs to ensure that every product labeled as identical is actually equivalent in its therapeutic and biological activity, (3) disruption of the traditional physician-patient relationship, and (4) lack of evidence that generic substitution produces cost savings to the consumer.

The 1974 report of the Office of Technology Assessment (OTA) on drug bioequivalence is reviewed. The OTA panel reported that "current standards and regulatory practices do not insure bioequivalency for drug products . . .". Since the Food and Drug Administration has not since issued regulations and standards for the listing of generic or chemical equivalents for pharmacology and bioavailability, equivalency cannot be assumed at this time. The 1975 position of the National Research Council's Drug Research Board, of supporting substitution in the absence of data indicating the substituted drug is not equivalent, is reviewed.

The discussion of this report emphasizes that important considerations concerning the moral and legal responsibilities of the physician for the patient's treatment were not included in the report. Finally, the responsibility of the physician to the patient is discussed in detail. Since the physician has the greater knowledge of the patient's past and current medical history and short and long-range therapeutic plan, only the physician should change a prescription.

References, 6.

CHEWNING, JOHN B. *Ohio State Medical Journal 71* (5):323-326, May 1975.

Savings from Generic Prescriptions. A Study of Thirty-Three Pharmacies in Rochester, New York

104 Brand name and generic prescriptions for 12 drugs were surveyed to determine the actual savings passed on to the consumer and the frequency with which generic prescriptions were dispensed with the brand name product. The thirty-three pharmacies surveyed included representatives of chain, independent, inner city and suburban pharmacies. The survey was conducted by actual shoppers who visited five to seven pharmacies to fill specific brand or generic prescriptions. Data on cost savings for each specific drug are presented. In general, generic prescriptions for ampicillin, erythromycin, propoxyphene and dioctyl sodium sulfosuccinate were filled at a lower price than comparable brand name prescriptions. Prescriptions for papaverine, pentaerythritol tetranitrate and conjugated estrogens were occasionally filled with a lower-priced generic product. No savings were available for penicillin V, chlorpheniramine, diphenylhydantoin, sulfisoxazole, or methenamine mandelate.

After the survey was completed, questionnaires were mailed to all pharmacists and each was additionally interviewed in order to assess the completeness of the first questionnaire; data and assessments from the interview were recorded on a second questionnaire. A sample of physicians at Strong Memorial Hospital and internists and family practitioners in the county also completed questionnaires. The pharmacists correctly identified a median of 18.5 drugs out of 22 drugs as having a generic alternative; the physicians identified a median of 14.1 drugs out of 22 drugs correctly. Specific data per drug for the "awareness of" and "stocking of" alternative products are presented. The data collected clearly indicated that "shopping around" for lower drug prices resulted in cost savings. An estimate of potential cost savings to the consumer for generic prescribing cannot be made on the basis of differences in listed wholesale cost between brand name and generic equivalents.

References, 31.

HORVITZ, RICHARD A.; MORGAN, JOHN P.; and FLECKENSTEIN, LAWRENCE. *Annals of Internal Medicine* 82 (5):601–607, May 1975.

A Quantitative Analysis of Antisubstitution Repeal

138 Prescription data from 20 Saskatchewan (Canada) pharmacies before and after the repeal of drug antisubstitution laws (January–June 1971 and January–June 1972) showed significant (0.05) increases in brand or generic substitution activity from 1.16 per cent to 3.08 per cent and in inpatient prescriptions, 4.61 per cent to 6.88 per cent. No significant differences were found in third-party prescriptions (16.54 per cent to 16.55 per cent) or in generic prescribing (9.80 per cent to 10.84 per cent).

In 1970, the Public Affairs Committee of the American Pharmaceutical Association sought repeal of state antisubstitution laws. Some states have responded, but not in sufficient numbers to examine the resulting patterns. Therefore, the study was done in Canada, where Saskatchewan became the fourth province to repeal antisubstitution laws on July 1, 1971. Physicians may indicate "no substitutes," but otherwise pharmacists can generically substitute across trade names without a formulary. Average patient charges for all prescriptions and for substituted prescriptions decreased slightly between 1971 and 1972. The average charge for generic prescriptions did not change, but the average charge for brand name (nonsubstituted) prescriptions increased from $3.56 to $4.81. However, the examination of prescriptions by unit price indicated a small price decrease over all prescriptions; a significant (0.05) price decrease for brand name (nonsubstituted) prescriptions (due, in part, to an increase in unit dispensed per prescription); a small price increase for generic prescriptions; and a significant (0.05) price increase for substituted prescriptions (partly confounded by the great change in quantity dispensed per prescription). The 1972 unit price for substituted drugs remained lower than the unit price for brand name drugs, although it was higher than for generic drugs. Results cannot be extrapolated to the United States should there be repeal of antisubstitution laws, but such studies should provide insight into the economic effects.

References, 10.

KOTZAN, JEFFREY, A.; HUNTER, ROBERT, H.; and TINDALL, WILLIAM, N. *Medical Marketing and Media 10* (5):18–20, May 1975.

The Michigan Generic Substitution Law: A Survey of Opinion

232

Many pharmacists and physicians regarded a Michigan law permitting generic substitution as generally confusing and one which would not result in cost savings to the consumer. The Michigan law was enacted in June 1974. In January 1975, prior to its scheduled April, 1975 date of effect, pharmacists and physicians (specialists, general practitioners and osteopaths) throughout the state were interviewed in person and by telephone. Some findings of the survey were: (1) A physician is permitted to write D.A.W. (dispense as written) on a prescription in order to prohibit generic substitution. One-half of the internists and 14 per cent of the pharmacists surveyed did not know the meaning of D.A.W. (2) One-third of the pharmacists and over one-half of the general practitioners reported that they did not completely understand the legislation. (3) Only a small percentage of the pharmacists felt that generic substitution would save the patient money. Most stated that the generic substitutes they would use were quality products and close in price to the brand name drugs. Many physicians felt there would be no cost savings because the pharmacist would charge the same even when he substituted. Pharmacists and physicians who felt prices would be lower disagreed as to whether the decrease in price would be noticeable. (4) Opinion differed as to the party with legal liability should an adverse reaction to a substitute drug occur. Overall, it was believed that pharmacists would most likely be held liable. Pharmacists were more likely than physicians to place the responsibility on the drug manufacturer.

References, 0.

STEWART, RAYMOND. *Medical Marketing and Media 10* (5):22–23, May 1975.

1974

PARCOST Comparative Drug Index

57

The objective of the PARCOST (prescriptions at reasonable cost) program is to assist the people of the province of Ontario in obtaining prescribed drug products of quality at reasonable cost by developing economies throughout the pharmaceutical industry and health professions. The program encourages fair competition and more efficient methods of distribution and utilization of pharmaceuticals made available through community pharmacies or hospitals.

The Comparative Drug Index lists prescription products by nature, strength, and dosage form of the active therapeutic ingredient. Comparable products are listed according to trade and/or nonproprietary name and supplier or manufacturer, and are arranged in order of relative maximum cost. Categories of similar drugs are printed on color-coded pages. The Index is intended to serve as a guide to practitioners in the identification of quality products, to pharmacists in the stocking of comparable products, and to professional committees in the selection of products for use in hospitals. Interchangeable pharmaceutical products are noted. Prices represent pharmacist costs from wholesalers; patient costs include a dispensing fee not to exceed $2.20. A 1972 survey found that 57 per cent of the prescriptions written in the province were done so with the intention of reducing patient costs. This is taken to indicate confidence in the list of interchangeable drug products.

References, 0. *Key words:* Maximum allowable cost.

DRUG QUALITY AND THERAPEUTICS COMMITTEE. Seventh Edition. Ottawa, Canada, Ministry of Health, 1974.

Generic Equivalency and FDA Approved Usage. What are the True Effects of Drugs?

81

Within the issue of generic equivalency, a major question is whether or not different brands of generically equivalent drugs yield a different effect on a patient's disease conditions or overall health condition. This paper examines the officially approved labeling of selected drugs. The labeling of different brands of a generic drug was examined with regard to indications, contraindications, warnings, precautions and adverse reactions. Within each of these major headings, the presence of various labeling items across the different brands was noted. The data revealed that for most of the generics in this study, the differences across various generics were quite large. The differences are considered separately in the paper, according to the generic name of each drug studied.

References, 0.

GIBSON, TYRONE. *Hospital Formulary Management 9* (*11*):39, 42, 44, 46, 48–49, 54, 56, 58, November 1974.

Consumer Price Differentials between Generic and Brand Name Prescriptions

91

The price per unit charged to consumers for generic prescriptions was significantly ($p < 0.05$) lower than the price per unit for brand name prescriptions for five out of seven common drugs at forty-five out of forty-six pharmacies.

Since the HEW Task Force on Prescription Drugs (1969) investigated differences between the acquisition cost of brand name and generic drugs to the pharmacist, the purpose of this study was to determine the price differential between generic and brand name prescriptions charged to the consumer. The seven generic drugs chosen for investigation were selected from the sixteen generic drugs contained in the Top 200 Drug List (R.A. Gosselin & Co., 1970) on the basis of their widespread availability and use and the presence of one or more brand name versions of the generic drug on the Top 200 Drug List. A sample of sixty pharmacies was randomly chosen for investigation. Forty-six pharmacies (23 independent and 23 chain) agreed to participate in the study. The prescription files of participating pharmacies were audited over a six-month period to determine the prescription prices paid by the consumer for both generic and brand name drugs.

The generic drug price was found to be significantly lower ($p < 0.05$) per unit for five drugs: tetracycline capsules 250 mg; meprobamate tablets 400 mg; reserpine tablets 0.25 mg; chloral hydrate capsules 500 mg; and penicillin G potassium tablets 400,000 units. The generic drug price was not significantly ($p < 0.05$) lower per unit for two drugs: digoxin tablets 0.25 mg and prednisone tablets 5 mg. Analysis of the data indicated that the average number of units in the generic and brand prescriptions was not significantly different. A second part of the study showed that the consumer price for all seven drugs at each pharmacy was not a factor of the operational characteristics (e.g., location, prescription pricing system) of the pharmacy. The authors concluded that the consumer price differential between generic and brand name prescriptions was a function of the differential in acquisition cost to the pharmacy.

References, 21.

GUMBHIR, ASHOK K.; and RODOWSKAS, CHRISTOPHER A., JR. *American Journal of Public Health* 64 (10):977–982, October 1974.

Equivalent Therapy at Lower Cost. The Oral Penicillins

122

An examination of list prices for branded and unbranded products of the oral penicillins revealed that: (1) generic prescribing does not necessarily result in lower prices and (2) generic prescribing does not ensure that the patient will pay the lowest price possible for equivalent therapy. The nature and effects of generic prescribing are discussed.

The authors list the therapeutic options available to a physician and the options available to the pharmacist who fills a generic prescription. The pharmacist can choose an unbranded or a branded product which is chemically identical to that prescribed, but there is no assurance that he will fill it with the lowest priced product. A list of the branded and unbranded products for each of the oral penicillins was compiled and the cost of equivalent therapy was computed for each. The data showed that marked cost differences can occur among equivalent therapeutic options. In order for a patient to receive the lowest priced generic equivalent, the authors recommend that the prescribing physician use both the generic or chemical name *and* specify the manufacturer or distributor. Unfortunately, the data necessary to compare list prices among both branded and unbranded products are generally not readily available to the physician.

References, 12.

KEMP, BERNARD A.; and MOYER, PAUL R. *Journal of the American Medical Association 228* (8):1009–1014, May 20, 1974.

Providing Quality Drugs Economically. The Role of State Formularies

157 The Tennessee Medicaid Drug Program is attempting to control costs by combining an "open-controlled" formulary with utilization review and bioequivalency evaluation. Before adopting the program, a survey was made of relevant studies and other states' experiences.

Formularies have been used to cut costs by decreasing inventories and recommending cheaper products. They are convenient for data processing and peer review. On the other hand, they may restrict the choice of therapy, require frequent revision and have administrative costs. Some simply list all agents by generic name to facilitate coding; other may restrict drugs, sources or both. Medical and economic judgement is involved and risk-benefit ratios must be weighed. Savings of up to $40 million a year from generic prescribing have been projected. However, the significance of inequivalent bioavailability of chemically equivalent products is controversial. Several recent studies question the availability of sufficient information for pharmacists to objectively evaluate competing products. States that have tried formularies that significantly restrict reimbursable drugs have not achieved the expected savings.

Not enough is known yet about those states that are attempting to encourage generic prescribing, though a Massachusetts survey suggests these efforts have been largely ineffective in altering prescribing habits. Several reports have indicated that programs which carefully monitor claims for abuses have cut costs significantly. Utilization surveillance with peer review may cut medical as well as drug costs by improving therapy. Based on available data, Tennessee decided to build into its program a relatively nonrestrictive formulary, a systematic review system and efforts to evaluate relative product efficacy. The formulary encompasses most prescribed drugs, with exceptions like over-the-counter drugs or anorectic drugs except in specified conditions. Price ceilings have been set for some dozen drugs at a calculated savings of over $400,000 a year. A contract was made with the University of Tennessee college of pharmacy for a bioavailability testing program for certain drugs, and eventually the formulary will include source limitations. Routine checks are made on drug utilization records for potential abuse by patients, prescribers or pharmacists. There are also renewal restrictions on all drugs. The program seems to be working efficiently—1973 cost per claim was only $4.29, professional fee included. It should also contribute important information on the significance of bioavailability problems.

References, 34. *Key words:* Drug utilization review.

MEYER, MARVIN C.; BATES, HERBERT, JR.; and SWIFT, ROBERT G. *Journal of the American Pharmaceutical Association NS14* (*12*):663–666, December 1974.

Physician Acceptance of Three Proposed Programs Designed to Reduce Prescription Prices

165

Physicians' perception of prescription drug prices as excessive was found to be significantly related to their receptivity to methods of reducing prescription drug prices by repeal of state antisubstitution laws, the use of a federal formulary or the use of a community formulary, and to their willingness to accept product selection by pharmacists if consumer price savings were assured.

A random sample of 500 physicians received a pretested mail questionnaire on university letterhead; the response rate was 64.6 per cent. On physicians' attitudes toward the average price paid by consumers for prescription drugs, 13.1 per cent believed that prescription drugs were a bargain for the value received, 36.1 per cent felt that they were priced about right for the value received, and 37.3 per cent thought that they were generally overpriced. Younger physicians and those in institutional practice tended to believe prescription drug prices were excessive. Physicians in large communities and those who were heavy prescribers tended to believe drug prices were about right or a bargain. Of those who believed drugs were overpriced, 51.5 per cent blamed drug manufacturers, 38.1 per cent blamed pharmacists and none blamed the prescribers themselves for excessive drug prices.

Earlier research is cited in which three-fourths of the private physicians surveyed said that they considered prices when prescribing, but few could estimate accurately (within 20 per cent) for their chosen drugs; estimates were consistently low. On the acceptance of pharmacists substituting less expensive chemically equivalent prescription drugs, 57.3 per cent indicated high acceptance; of those who believed prices were excessive, 76.3 per cent indicated high acceptance. On their attitude toward a federal formulary, 25 per cent indicated acceptance; of those who believed prices were excessive, 37.5 per cent indicated acceptance. On attitudes toward a community formulary, 32.1 per cent indicated acceptance; of those who believed prices were excessive, 43.0 per cent indicated acceptance. On attitudes toward repeal of antisubstitution laws, 27.6 per cent were in favor; of those who believed prices were excessive, 40.6 per cent were in favor. Efforts should be made to provide price information to physicians.

References, 23. *Key words:* Maximum allowable cost.

NELSON, ARTHUR A.; and GAGNON, JEAN P. *Drugs in Health Care 1* (*1*):27–37, Summer 1974.

Drug Bioequivalence

169 This report, prepared for the United States Senate Committee on Labor and Public Welfare, examines the relationship between chemical and therapeutic equivalence of drug products (tablets and capsules) and assesses the capability of current technology to determine whether drug products with the same physical and chemical composition produce comparable therapeutic effects. Chemically equivalent drug products which produce clinically important and measurable differences in therapeutic effect differ in "bioavailability." (Drug products which are not chemically equivalent but which produce the same therapeutic effect are referred to as pharmaceutical "alternatives"; they are not chemical or pharmaceutical "equivalents.") The report concludes that current standards and regulatory practices do not insure bioequivalence. Variations in bioavailability have been recognized as being responsible for a few therapeutic failures. The technology is available for bioavailability studies, but it is not feasible to conduct such studies for all drugs. Drug classes for which evidence of bioequivalence is critical should be identified, based on clinical importance, ratio of therapeutic to toxic concentration in the blood and pharmaceutical characteristics. New standards for quality and uniform bioavailability of new drug products should be developed and continually revised. Laws requiring manufacturers to maintain and make records on bioavailability tests available to the FDA should be strengthened. Pre-1962 exemptions to drug quality standards should be eliminated. The *United States Pharmacopeia* and the *National Formulary* should be replaced by a single federal organization to set standards. An official list of interchangeable drug products should be established. A seven-page bibliography is included with the report.

References, 80.

OFFICE OF TECHNOLOGY ASSESSMENT. Washington, D.C., United States Government Printing Office, 1974.

Prescribing Patterns in the New York City Medicaid Program

187 A sample of 5,271 prescription orders for both prescription and over-the-counter (OTC) drugs submitted to the New York City (NYC) Medicaid program was analyzed by therapeutic category. The cost of medication by category and the frequency of generic prescriptions by category was determined. The sample consisted of prescriptions on every fifth invoice submitted on May 20, 1971. Drugs prescribed were categorized into sixteen therapeutic classes according to the formulary of the American Society of Hospital Pharmacists. The most frequently prescribed classes of drugs were central nervous system drugs (21.1 per cent), systemic anti-infectives (15.7 per cent) and antihistamines (8.1 per cent).

The physician has the option under the Medicaid program to prescribe by generic name or by brand name. Among prescription drugs, generic prescribing was most frequent for cardiovascular drugs (41 per cent), anti-infectives (23 per cent) and spasmolytic agents (18 per cent). Great variation in the frequency of generic prescribing existed among the subcategories of each drug category. Overall, an average of 13 per cent of drug orders for prescription drugs were written by generic name. Generic prescriptions for OTC drugs were for single or multiple vitamin products. A comparison with prescribing patterns found in other studies revealed no significant differences for most categories. Specific areas of difference could be explained by the nature of health care services for the NYC Medicaid population.

Cost analysis of the sample prescription orders indicated that the average price of prescription drugs was $4.24 and of OTC drugs $2.06, for an average of $3.79 for all medications. This compares favorably with the "average prescription price" (unspecified as to prescription or OTC medications) of $3.92 determined in a 1971 survey by *American Druggist.* The paper concludes with a general discussion on cost savings due to generic prescribing.

References, 17. *Key words:* Drug utilization review.

ROSENBERG, STEPHEN N.; BERENSON, LOUISE B.; KAVALER, FLORENCE; and GORELIK, ELIHU A. *Medical Care* 12 (2):138–151, February 1974.

The Drug Business in the Context of Canadian Health Care Programs

204

Public health programs providing hospital and physician care are available to Canadians and are financed by tax revenues. Outpatient prescription drugs are thus the only health care expense the individual must absorb, and this has received a great deal of attention. At the retail level, much has been done to keep prescription drug prices from skyrocketing. In an effort to aid this measure, the federal government has attempted to encourage generic rather than brand name prescribing and they have also intervened in the areas of quality control and retail pricing with a high degree of success. A scheme providing drug benefits is imminent, whether in conjunction with the Canadian government or as an independent venture on the part of some provinces. Perhaps a cost sharing health program on a federal-provincial level will be instituted.

References, 6.

RUDERMAN, A. PETER. *International Journal of Health Services* 4 (4):641–650, 1974.

Drug Antisubstitution Studies. I: Estimation of Possible Savings by Repeal of Antisubstitution Laws

235

This study indicates that 3.1–4.6 per cent of total drug costs could be saved by generic substitution. Two levels of savings were determined: savings over the wholesale purchase of the prescribed product (4.6 per cent) and savings over direct purchase from the manufacturer of the prescribed product (3.1 per cent). Data on prescription volume, retail volume, pharmacists' acquisition costs and prescription size were collected from source books for the one hundred most frequently prescribed (accounting for 50.5 per cent of prescriptions) drug products in the United States in 1971. The study was based solely on drug costs and did not take into consideration possible quality differences in the products nor administrative costs which could be inherent to any generic prescription program. The findings of the current study were compared with the conclusion of the HEW Task Force on Prescription Drugs (1971), that 5–8 per cent of drug costs could be saved through a generic prescription program.

Several differences in the methodology of the two studies which could account for the different conclusions are: (1) the current study was stricter in its requirements for drug substitution, (2) arithmetic errors were found in the Task Force report, (3) the Task Force study applied only to products used by persons age 65 and over, and thus included more maintenance drugs, and (4) the Task Force study was conducted on 409 drug products, accounting for 88 per cent of all prescriptions dispensed. Since more drugs with no generic equivalent were included in the current study, the results may be an underestimate of the percentage savings on all drugs. Finally, since only 25 per cent of drug purchases appear to be direct purchases, the true savings are probably closer to 4.6 per cent of all drug costs than 3.1 per cent, leading the authors to conclude that at least 4 per cent of the total drug costs could be saved by generic substitution. In 1971, this savings would have equaled $224 million.

References, 8.

STROM, BRIAN L.; STOLLEY, PAUL D.; and BROWN, TORREY C. *Drugs in Health Care I* (2):99–103, Fall 1974.

Drug Antisubstitution Studies. II: Evaluation of Pharmacists' Attitudes Toward Repeal of Antisubstitution Laws

236

Pharmacists' attitudes toward drug substitution were evaluated by determining their degree of substitution where it was legally permitted. The State of Maryland had recently enacted a partial repeal of its antisubstitution law, and the article discussed the new law and analyzed what future changes in the law might maximize the participation of the pharmacist. Questionnaires were mailed to a sample of pharmacies throughout the state and to the Directors of Pharmaceutical Services of every chain of pharmacies in the state. Due to the poor response of chain pharmacies, the chain data were not analyzed. Seventy per cent (161 of 231) of the individual pharmacies responded. Twenty per cent of respondents wanted the new substitution law to be repealed entirely, either due to objections over specific provisions in it or due to philosophic disagreement with the idea of substitution.

Five reasons for not participating in substitution were determined: the state requirement that the prescriber be notified in writing of substitution; doubts about drug product equivalence; fears of legal liability; state requirement that all savings be passed on to the consumer; and a general negative attitude toward substitution. The requirement for written notification was the major obstacle to participation by the pharmacist, with 82 per cent of respondents wanting a change in the law, either to oral notification or to none at all. An educational campaign about substitution is recommended as a way of dispelling doubts about liability and drug equivalence.

References, 1.

STROM, BRIAN L.; STOLLEY, PAUL D.; and BROWN, TORREY C. *Drugs in Health Care 1* (2):104–107, Fall 1974.

1973

Consumers' Guide to Prescription Prices

90

Information on reading a prescription is offered. A listing of average retail prices for brand name, generic and some over-the-counter drug products is provided and information included on form, strength, prescription size and disease or condition the drug product is commonly used to treat.

This is a trade paperback and not part of the professional literature. It does not provide information on how the particular drugs in the price list were selected, nor does it attempt to distinguish generic from brand name drugs—this leads to considerable confusion when trying to find information on a particular drug product.

References, 0.

GULICK, WILLIAM. Syracuse, Consumer Age Press, 1973.

Trade Names or Proper Names? A Problem for the Prescriber

106

A 1973 London symposium on prescribing by trade or generic name, attended by representatives of the pharmaceutical industry, pharmacists and medical practitioners, offered suggestions on the problem of drug substitution in the absence of therapeutic equivalence.

In National Health Service Hospitals, pharmacists may substitute alternative brands of a drug product; this is thought to reduce both costs and processing time. Buying fewer drug products in bulk yielded savings amounting to approximately one per cent of the total National Health Service drug budget. Outside the hospital setting, substitution by pharmacists is not permitted. Variation in the effects of different formulations of the same drug has been found. The pharmaceutical industry encourages brand name prescribing as a way of recovering research and development costs. Pharmacists prefer brand names because these drugs are more profitable and because there are differences between brands of drug products containing the same active ingredient. Also, pharmacists are unfamiliar with patient histories. Most general practitioners prescribe by brand name because they usually lack the time to study clinical trials reports, and become familiar with drug products only through advertising. Researchers argue that generic names convey more information about active ingredients (especially important with combination antibiotics) and facilitate communication among medical personnel. Nurses request that whichever prescribing system is chosen, it be standardized. For therapeutic equivalence to be demonstrated, the correct quantity of the active ingredient and the fact that it reaches the site of action, must be established. It has been shown that formulation can affect absorption (bioavailability), especially with combination products. A National Pharmaceutical Laboratory to set drug standards was proposed.

References, 4. *Key words:* Inpatient settings.

HUSKISSON, E.C. *British Medical Journal* 4 (5886):225–228, October 27, 1973.

The Peril of "Non-Peer Peer Review"

146 I am very concerned about Senator Kennedy's call for "peer review" of physicians by pharmacists at the American Pharmaceutical Association Annual Meeting in July 1973. I do not see how the pharmacist, with his typical 4-year (sic) college degree, can challenge the judgment of a physician who has prepared intensively for 12 or more years. The pharmacist has no patient history, is not knowledgeable about allergies and knows nothing about the physician's rationale and differential diagnosis. His review could even be construed as the unlawful practice of medicine. Senator Kennedy proposes that pharmacists give instructions on how to take prescribed medicines, but I am sure most physicians already do this. The physician chooses a drug brand for good reasons. Pharmacist substitution would not take into account such factors as lack of generic equivalency, bioavailability, allergies and previous experience with the individual patient. A lower price could lead to an adverse drug reaction. The answer to Senator Kennedy's rhetorical question about why more than one pharmaceutical house should make the same product is simple—free competition. It is misrepresentation to pick the highest list price for a brand name to compare with the lowest catalog price of a generic drug. The Senator's charge that the drug industry makes excessive profits ignores the time, research and money that goes into developing new drugs, some of which will "flop." It is too bad that the busy physician has little time to study pharmacology, but continuing medical education, publications and first-rate advertising will have to help him keep abreast. In conclusion, physicians will have to rebut any legislation that misrepresents our professional situation and will interfere with delivery of the best medical care.

References, 0. *Key words:* Drug utilization review.

LEES, WILLIAM M. *Illinois Medical Journal 144* (*6*):597–598, December 1973.

Multiple Brands of Prescription Drugs: Effects and Implications for Pharmacy Inventories

175 Results of a national study conducted by the Lea-Mendota Research Group of Lea, Inc. for the Pharmaceutical Manufacturers Association show little or no grounds for fears that the introduction of multiple brands of drugs seriously affects the size and cost of pharmacy inventories. The recent increase in competitive branded products stems largely from difficulties in introducing new entities, plus the expiration of patents on therapeutically important products. A representative sample of retail pharmacies listed which products they had on hand to fill generically written prescriptions for 10 drug forms, which represent almost half of these prescriptions. They included three products most frequently alleged to be inventory problems—ampicillin, tetracycline and penicillin G potassium. There were slight regional differences, and mean inventory level increased somewhat with number of new prescriptions. Differences by urban, suburban, or rural location were insignificant. Stores belonging to larger chains stocked a slightly larger inventory. Nearly 80 per cent of the pharmacists, if presented with a prescription for a specific brand of ampicillin which either is not normally stocked or happens to be

out-of-stock, would call the physician for permission to substitute, or borrow from another pharmacy. The average number of such calls to physicians during the preceding month was 2. Most seem to manage their ampicillin inventories by stocking only products likely to be prescribed in their area and being able to readily obtain products not in stock.

Almost 70 per cent said they could get same day delivery from wholesalers. When asked what circumstances, other than an out-of-stock situation, would induce them to recommend an alternate brand of ampicillin, only 2 per cent checked size of inventory and almost 40 per cent responded "no circumstances." Only 4 per cent saw the stocking of multiple products as their most serious problem. The majority did not even see it as a difficult problem. The advent of multiple brand competition has resulted in substantial price declines, suggesting that pharmacist investment in inventories has not increased despite the availability of more products. *Lilly Digest* figures seem to support this. The trend toward increases in multisource products will undoubtedly continue. The findings of this study demonstrate that this phenomenon has not required larger inventories or increased overall inventory expense. The price competition fostered provides benefits to both pharmacists and patients.

References, 0.

PHARMACEUTICAL MANUFACTURERS ASSOCIATION. Washington, D.C., The Association, July 1973.

How Cost Effective are Generics?

258

Blue Cross called upon the Pennsylvania Insurance Commission (PIC) to study cost differences between generic and brand name drugs. A study was designed to determine the validity of PIC's conclusion that if generic prescribing were the norm, a savings of between 60–95 per cent would result. It would also determine the effect of this savings on the payment for drugs to hospitals.

A stratified sample which included 20 per cent of the 95 hospitals in Western Pennsylvania was classified into five categories according to daily census. A tabulation was then made of each prescription filled by the pharmacy service within a 24-hour period. Data included name, strength, quantity and drug cost to the hospital. In all hospitals included in the study, more than half of the drugs prescribed were purchased at the lowest *Red Book* price. Twenty-five per cent of the drugs prescribed were obtained at prices below the *Red Book* figure. It appears that, as a result of bulk purchase or membership in a group purchasing plan, hospital pharmacies can purchase drugs at a cost lower than the lowest *Red Book* price and thus save $700,000 above the savings secured through *Red Book* purchasing. Savings through purchase of generic equivalents saves only 3.5 per cent of total drug costs, or about $600,000 for the area. This falls well below the projected 60–95 per cent savings. Thus, requiring generic prescribing would have little effect. The only way to secure a substantial decrease in drug costs to hospitals would be through a national quality testing program which would cut $42 million. A revision of the inefficient drug purchasing plans already existing would also be helpful.

References, 4.

WOLFE, HARVEY. *Hospitals* 47 (9):100, 104, 106, 108, May 1, 1973.

1972

Product Selection: Community Formularies and Legal Aspects

118 Dr. Kanig argues that the entire burden of selection of drug products for generic substitution should not be placed onto the pharmacist alone. He advocates a system wherein a formulary is established on a state or national level which contains drug products which were judged to be equivalent by a council of experts, based on their evaluation of relevant clinical and biological data. The pharmacist could substitute generically within the formulary if he desired and would be required to do so if requested by the patient. This view of the pharmacist's role in product selection is thus opposite to that of the American Pharmaceutical Association, which stated in its 1971 "White Paper" that ". . . the pharmacist would also assume the responsibility for determining that the substituted product is as effective therapeutically as the one prescribed." While Dr. Kanig agrees that the pharmacist is indeed the only drug expert on the health care team, he feels that being an expert does not enable one to make judgments on biological equivalence among several drug products allegedly equivalent. The concept of Good Manufacturing Practices, in which all aspects of the procedures used in producing drug products are controlled, and its impact on generic substitution is discussed. The Kentucky formulary system, upon which the advocated model system is based, is described.

References, 0.

KANIG, JOSEPH L. *American Journal of Pharmacy* 144 (5):133–138, September–October, 1972.

Pharmacists' and Physicians' Attitudes Toward Removal of the Prohibition on Brand Substitution: A Comparative Study

155 A study was conducted to determine which characteristics of pharmacists and physicians and which issues were significant in influencing attitudes concerning the removal of the ban on brand substitution.

Questionnaires were mailed to 600 pharmacists and 600 physicians practicing in Wisconsin and of these 58.5 per cent and 59.3 per cent, respectively, responded. Among the results of this study, which should not be projected outside Wisconsin, neither age nor sex were statistically significant in pharmacist opinion on removal of the ban; among physicians, however, age was a factor since 52 per cent of those under 40 favored removal of the restrictions. The percentage decreased as age increased. No significance was shown in relating community size to attitudes on the issue or in correlating pharmacist status to opinions on removal of the prohibition.

While this study indicates that neither group has a majority view on either side of the issue, it is significant that 40 per cent of the responding physicians favored removal of the ban. Findings also suggest that members of the American Pharmaceutical Association were more likely to support that organization's position on the issue than were nonmembers. Eighty per cent of physicians responding favored the use of a hospital formulary system which would allow pharmacists to substitute within the hospital setting and more than 635 favored the same privilege for community pharmacists. Numerous other results are reported. Removing the antisubstitution laws would remove the state as a decision maker in the prescribing and dispensing of medicines, but in its place would come formulary boards which would set limitations. Economic sanctions would impose further restrictions on the pharmacist which would prevent him from exercising his professional judgment.

References, 38.

McCORMICK, WILLIAM C.; and HAMMEL, ROBERT W. *Medical Marketing and Media* 7 (*10*):27–30, 35–37, October 1972.

Controlling Drug Costs

162

Research indicating that drug costs could be reduced by substituting generic or similar items of frequently prescribed drugs suggests several ways of controlling drug expenditures. Data from a mid-Atlantic county of 112,000 people in 1968 showed aggregate savings of $34,709 by substituting similarly acting drugs and $22,931 by substituting generic equivalents for some of the 20 most frequently prescribed drugs. Average prescription prices are presented for 11 drugs and their substitutes.

Thus, reducing costs on just a small number of widely prescribed drug products will result in considerable savings in a health insurance program. Other suggestions for reducing drug costs—and improving the quality of prescribing—include (1) standards for drug manufacturers such that physicians will be more willing to prescribe generic products, (2) shorter patent periods for drugs, (3) continuing education and relicensing programs, especially for older physicians, to assure appropriate prescribing, (4) withdrawal of worthless drugs and higher standards of effectiveness for introducing new drugs, (5) limiting health insurance coverage on products used without specific indication (for example, tranquilizers), and (6) formularies and utilization review programs.

References, 1. *Key words:* Drug utilization review, formularies.

MULLER, CHARLOTTE; STOLLEY, PAUL D.; and BECKER, MARSHALL H. *American Journal of Public Health* 62 (*6*):755–756, June 1972.

1971

White Paper on the Pharmacist's Role in Product Selection

2

An overview of antisubstitution laws and of the position of the American Pharmaceutical Association is provided; the Association advocates the amendment of these laws to allow pharmacists to select the source of multisource drug products prescribed by trade name alone. This achieves many of the goals of generic prescribing and accounts for approximately 10 per cent of the market; this percentage is expected to increase as patents expire and more single source drug products become multisource products. The amendment of the laws should decrease consumer drug costs, increase the efficiency of health personnel and of drug product marketing and should not adversely affect the physician-patient relationship. The paper discusses therapeutic, professional, legal and economic issues, and reviews the roles of the professional associations of health practitioners. It reprints the February 20, 1971 testimony of the FDA commissioner (before the Senate Subcommittee on Monopoly) on the quality, effectiveness and safety of United States pharmaceutical products. On economic issues, the paper notes that pharmacists could reduce their inventory of multisource products and stock the lowest cost product of acceptable quality, thus reducing wholesale and operating costs. The HEW Task Force on Prescription Drugs study and the cost savings in using low-cost chemical equivalents of 409 of the most frequently prescribed drugs for the elderly are discussed, as is the pharmaceutical industry's opposition to the American Pharmaceutical Association's position on antisubstitution laws.

References, 0.

AMERICAN PHARMACEUTICAL ASSOCIATION. Washington, D.C., The Association, 1971.

Drug Substitutions

6

This article elucidates the American Medical Association's position on the repeal of the antisubstitution laws and on hospital formularies. The negative feelings concerning the repeal of these laws are not in contradiction of the support of hospital formularies. The hospital formulary system does not provide blanket authorization for dispensing a nonproprietary drug or a proprietary drug different to the one prescribed. However, it does allow the physician to use his discretion and professional judgment at the time of prescribing, to approve or disapprove the dispensing of a nonproprietary drug or a proprietary drug other than that prescribed. Opposition to the repeal of the law is based on the premise that blanket delegation of the privilege to substitute would remove the physician's right to exercise his medical judgment. With the implementation of the hospital formulary, this privilege is insured.

References, 0.

ANONYMOUS. *Hospital Formulary Management* 6 (12):29, December 1971.

Role of the Compendia in Controlling Factors Affecting Bioavailability of Drug Products

23

The role of the *United States Pharmacopeia* and the *National Formulary* in establishing standards for controlling factors affecting the bioavailability of drug products is discussed. The two works here cited serve as the official compendia and contain standards for the strength, quality and purity of drugs. Since drugs are combined with nontherapeutic agents to create a drug product in various dosage forms, there is a need to establish the equivalency or nonequivalency of the drug. Thus, certain factors may affect the therapeutic efficacy of the dosage form employed. A tripartite structure involving the FDA, the manufacturer and the pharmacist provide a system of checks and balances in order to assure that the public receives only top quality drugs and drug products. The official compendia, revised every five years by field specialists, bases admission on the therapeutic value of the drug. Those drugs which comply with compendial standards meet with chemical equivalency but not necessarily biological or clinical equivalency; however, it is rare for a drug to meet compendial standards and not produce the desired clinical effect. Nonetheless, the establishment of additional standards and specifications would assure clinical equivalency of drug products. A number of factors affect the therapeutic activity of a drug: isomeric form, tablet disintegration test, crystalline modification, particle size, hydrates, chemical form, dissolution test, manufacturing and formulation factors and other factors such as variations within the same batch. Most are controlled by already existing standards, but the compendia are aware of the need to establish test procedures to evaluate the bioavailability of drug products. Ideally these tests should be carried out on humans but that is impractical for medical, economic and other reasons. At present the dissolution test is the only method of quantifying the bioavailability of drugs, but new improvements are seen in the future.

References, 22.

BLAKE, MARTIN I. *Journal of the American Pharmaceutical Association NS 11 (11)*:603–611, November 1971.

Brands, Generics, Prices and Quality: The Prescribing Debate after a Decade

174

This review contains chapters on economics, therapeutics, the roles of the *United States Pharmacopeia,* the *National Formulary* and FDA, government procurement programs, the recommendations of the Pharmaceutical Manufacturers Association, and a chronology of events supporting the contention that equality among generic drug products must be demonstrated not assumed. The issue of how physicians ought to write prescriptions and how pharmacists should dispense them is reviewed. In particular the report considers whether significant savings result from generic prescribing. It notes that the professions are increasingly careful to select products from firms they "know and trust," and that there is no evidence to support the idea that generic prescribing and dispensing result in significantly lower overall prices (cites the 1967 American Medical Association survey and 1969 HEW Task Force on Prescription Drugs report). Medicaid/Medicare are referred to as "financial calamities." The report considers the literature on biopharmaceutics and the relationship of generic prescribing to drug quality. It discusses national drug laws, official standards and the role of the FDA, but stresses reliance on responsible manufacturers for assistance in assuring drug quality. It notes that the guideline in federal drug purchasing is economy-plus-quality, not blanket generic prescribing. The conclusions are that there is a need for improvement in manufacturing standards and the Association encourages informed judgment by health professionals in prescribing but notes that the costs of manufacturing, marketing and research must be recognized.

References, not counted; footnotes used.

PHARMACEUTICAL MANUFACTURERS ASSOCIATION. Washington, D.C., The Association, 1971.

1970

The New Handbook of Prescription Drugs: Official Names, Prices, and Sources for Patient and Doctor

36

This handbook discusses the characteristics of the drug industry; drug product testing and safety; relationships among the drug industry, physicians and medical schools and the consequent ethical problems; rational prescribing; generic versus brand name drugs and their relationship to unnecessary expenditures of Medicaid/Medicare funds; and the need for a national drug label law. It reviews approximately 60 basic drugs used to treat more than 90 per cent of adult outpatients. The bulk of the book is an alphabetical prescription drug list (brand name cross-referenced with generic name) offering commentary, and active ingredients and amounts in each dosage unit. Comparative prices are included for each manufacturer of a particular drug product. Appendices cover prescribing for children, the top 200 drugs in 1967 and the addresses of some distributors of generic drugs.

References, not counted; footnotes used.

BURACK, RICHARD. New York, Ballantine Books, 1970.

1969

The Cost of Drugs

5

The strong emotional reaction to the subject of drug costs ignores the fact that, according to the recent report of a subcommittee of the Public Expenditure Committee, costs rose from just 0.3 per cent to 0.5 per cent of New Zealand's gross national product between 1946–47 and 1967–68. The Walsh Committee pointed out the difficulties of determining whether the consumer gets good value for money, but decreases in general hospital bed use and duration of stay in mental hospitals imply benefits from improved medical care. Even though the country can clearly afford its drugs, they are expensive enough to warrant concern with cost control.

There can be little argument with the Committee's recommendations that proper education in prescribing is basic and that there should be more facilities to ensure the purity and efficacy of domestic and imported drugs.

Some Committee suggestions, such as abolishing brand names and permitting hospital boards to purchase drugs patented in New Zealand from nonpatented sources, are too simplistic. Many factors are involved in drug efficacy. The branded products of reputable firms are subjected to quality control and drugs from nonpatented sources should at least have to submit evidence of their clinical effectiveness. A *British Medical Journal* editorial supported the retention of brand names. The House of Commons decided against abolishing them because of international trade implications and opposed disregarding patents in purchases for the National Health Service. Incidentally, lack of patent protection is considered responsible for the Italian drug industry's notable lack of innovation and high prices. The Public Expenditure Committee has recommended setting up an independent Medicines

Commission to be responsible for licensing drugs to be sold in New Zealand, providing information to doctors, conducting research and planning on drug control, and advising the Government on medicines. Evolution is inevitable but radical changes and bureaucratic burdens that could stifle a system that has served so well must be avoided.

References, 3. *Key words:* Patents and prices

ANONYMOUS. *New Zealand Medical Journal 69* (440):33–34, January 1969.

White Paper on the Therapeutic Equivalence of Chemically Equivalent Drugs

41

The therapeutic equivalence of equal doses of chemically equivalent drugs produced by different manufacturers cannot be assumed. Also, there are usually no data available on the biological activity of chemically equivalent drugs other than those provided by the manufacturer in filing a New Drug Application. This report, by a subcommittee of the Policy Advisory Committee of the Drug Efficacy Study, prepared an addendum on the problem which was forwarded to the FDA. The more potent a drug, the greater the need for proof of therapeutic equivalence. This proof may require in vivo tests of each formulation of a drug or even each lot of each formulation. However, in vitro tests might be substituted in cases where blood levels provide an index of therapeutic activity. Large scale human subject testing imposes an unacceptable burden on drug manufacturers. One solution is to require manufacturers to submit evidence of composition, purity and quality, plus data on disintegration, dispersion and dissolution rates and from other tests, to demonstrate both chemical and biological equivalence. If in vitro or animal tests do not correlate with the effects in humans, clinical tests should be required. If better standards and test procedures for establishing therapeutic equivalence are put into effect, generic prescribing may become more widespread.

References, 0.

CASTLE, W.B.; ASTWOOD, E.B.; FINLAND, MAXWELL; and KEEFER, CHESTER S. *Journal of the American Medical Association 208* (7):1171–1172, May 19, 1969.

Generic Terminology and the Cost of Drugs

70

Lowering the price of drugs to the patient has recently become an issue of concern to physicians, legislators and laymen, and views on how this can be accomplished are discussed. To combat higher drug costs, a limited effort has been made, with successful results, to require the use of the generic name on the prescription.

To be marketed, a drug must meet the standards of the *United States Pharmacopeia* or the *National Formulary* or conform to FDA regulations. Those which do not measure up can be removed from the market. While legislators agree that purchase of a drug by its generic name will result in lower prices, it appears too that generic drugs can be as safe as trade name drugs. Physician concern lies with seeing that the patient receives the drug of highest quality and effectiveness at the least cost to him. Since not all manufactured drugs are of like quality due to various factors mentioned which can affect the clinical behavior of the drug, physicians tend to choose drugs from reputable manufacturers. The cost factor, however, is the responsibility of the pharmacist, who may get the drug at a lower price but not pass that reduction onto the consumer, due to his fee or markup.

The conclusion offered is that purchasing from a quality manufacturer—one who meets required standards, has technical capability, exerts sufficient controls and charges less for his product—would, along with the use of generic terminology, result in the lowering of drug costs to the consumer.

References, 9.

FRIEND, DALE G.; GOOLKASIAN, A. RICHARDSON; HASSAN, WILLIAM E., JR.; and VONA, JOSEPH P. *Journal of the American Medical Association 209* (*1*):80–84, July 7, 1969.

Cross-References

For further information on substitution, see:

ABSTRACT NUMBER	PAGE NUMBER	ABSTRACT NUMBER	PAGE NUMBER
18	57	161	213
26	54	176	79
49	13	177	35
58	34	201	196
71	28	216	32
120	48	242	52
152	216	244	50
160	29	246	152

IX

Drug Cost Controls: Patent Restrictions, Negotiated Prices

Fundamental changes in patent policy toward drugs have been proposed in order to increase competition and lower drug costs. Some programs controlling a substantial volume of prescriptions obtain cost savings by negotiating product costs directly with suppliers.
Key words: Patents and prices.

1976

California's Volume Purchase Plan

4

The background and components of California's Volume Purchase Plan (VPP) are discussed. Included are an editorial, negative comments from pharmacists throughout the state, a discussion of how the plan is "handcuffing" the pharmacist, letters from state wholesalers suggesting that VPP will not work as proposed, unfavorable comments from state pharmacy, educational and medical associations and institutions, and a report from the Pharmaceutical Manufacturers Association against the plan. Objections are that the plan interferes with private enterprise, that the professional fee for dispensing drugs is inadequate, and that maintaining separate inventories for VPP drug products is difficult and costly.

In brief, VPP would allow the state to bid with manufacturers for annual requirements of the 150 largest volume prescription drug items, totaling approximately 70 per cent of the expenditures for outpatient drugs under Medi-Cal. The products would be distributed to pharmacies through normal wholesale channels. Each pharmacy would receive a 3-month supply at no charge. The pharmacy would receive only a professional fee for drugs dispensed under the program; for drugs not included in the program, the pharmacy would receive a professional fee plus state allowances under other programs. It is suggested that under VPP the state maintains control over both drug quality and management (the latter through computer monitoring). The start-up date was to have been May 1, 1977, but the program has been abandoned.

References, 0.

ANONYMOUS. *Pharmacy West,* February 1976.

1970

Drug Patents, Compulsory Licenses, Prices and Innovation

68

United States patent and licensing provisions and similar laws in other countries, especially the United Kingdom are reviewed. Special requirements for inventions relating to food and medicine are noted and government hearings on patent protection and proposals to reduce patent terms on drugs from 17 to 3 years are discussed. Compulsory licensing and its relationship to market forces is examined. Investment in research and development increases when there is a chance of realizing a new product that will be protected from unlicensed imitations for a period of time sufficient to recoup investment funds. The average research and development time is 8 years for a new product, and is increasing as government drug clearance and approval requirements become more stringent. A 1962 survey of 30 corporations found that 25 of them allocate 15–75 per cent more funds to research and development than they would if there were no prospect of obtaining full-term patents. Cases illustrating positive and negative effects of compulsory licensing are presented. The author notes that the tendency of government agencies to take title to inventions arising from federally-funded research is discouraging to potential researchers and suggests that charges of excessive profits in the pharmaceutical industry are unjustified.

References, 0.

A commentary by Frederick M. Scherer suggests that Forman is affected by "subjective perception." Scherer discusses his own survey (around 1959) of 91 American corporations which found that 52 per cent of them said that their research and development progress would be unaffected by compulsory licensing. He argues that the patent system slows innovation, as do image advantages and factors such as managerial experience or unique distribution channels. He proposes compulsory licensing of drug patents, beginning three years after FDA approval of full-scale introduction of the product on the market.

References, 0.

A commentary by William W. Eaton suggests that the patent system stimulates invention and creativity and that widespread compulsory licensing will destroy the basics of the patent system. Eaton maintains that the drug industry and the medical profession should work together to provide information to the public about the drug scene.

References, 0.

A commentary by Leonard G. Schifrin suggests that prices are reasonable if they cover the costs of efficiently bringing forth products and making them available to consumers and if the prices also provide a profit level that justifies investment and risk taking in drug innovation and manufacture. Schifrin endorses a three-year exclusivity period followed by compulsory licensing.

References, 0.

A commentary by Rosalind Schulman discusses the need for more flexibility in licensing and for the collection and analysis of relevant statistics. She offers data on products marketed, on company profits and on return on investment for the drug industry versus all manufacturing.

References, 3.

FORMAN, HOWARD I. *In* Cooper, Joseph D., Editor. *Economics of Drug Innovation.* Proceedings of the First Seminar on Economics of Pharmaceutical Innovation, April 1969. Washington, D.C., American University, 1970. Pages 177–198.

Cross-References

For further information on patents and prices, see:

ABSTRACT NUMBER	PAGE NUMBER	ABSTRACT NUMBER	PAGE NUMBER
5	142	43	54
18	57	208	22
34	125	216	32

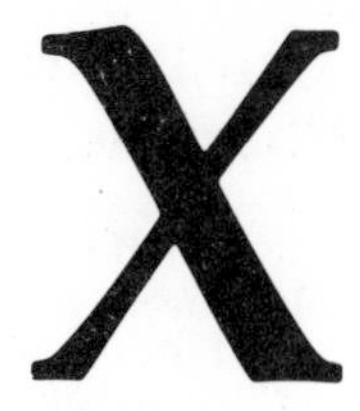

Dispensing Cost Controls: Pharmacist Reimbursement

The cost of ingredients is only a part of the price of the average prescription; the remainder provides for dispensing services, overhead expenses, and profit. Devising sound methods for determining equitable reimbursement levels for pharmaceutical services has become a key issue in cost containment efforts. Key word: Reimbursement.

1977

The Mysteries of Prescription Pricing in Retail Pharmacies

21

This study involved a two-week sample of retail drug prices from 20 pharmacies in a large midwestern city. A review of more than 13,000 prescriptions for 100 representative drug products revealed substantial price variations among pharmacies and within the same pharmacy for the study period. These unpredictable pricing practices serve to discourage rational purchasing behavior on the part of consumers. For example, prices for 25 tetracycline hydrochloride 250 mg ranged from $1.37 to $4.51. Differences in markup could account for this interpharmacy price variation. The highest percentage markup among the 15 most frequently prescribed drugs was 92.8 per cent for erythromycin 250 mg. Within the same pharmacy, prices for the identical prescription varied as much as 130 per cent. With one exception, it was not possible to classify the pharmacies as consistently low or high in drug prices. The data do not support the suggestion that the price variation can be explained by self-paying versus insured consumers.

References, 7.

BERKI, S.E.; RICHARDS, J.W.; and WEEKS, H.A. *Medical Care 15* (3):241–250, March 1977.

Third Party Reimbursement for Clinical Pharmacy Services: Philosophy and Practice

167 The operation of the Ohio State University Hospitals program of third-party reimbursement for professional services of the pharmacist is detailed. The program's concept is unique in that the clinical services eligible for reimbursement are not associated with drug costs. The program is guided by a patient care philosophy which focuses on the patient's health and satisfaction.

Seven steps required to obtain reimbursement are outlined. (1) a total commitment to the patient's health needs by hospital pharmacy management, (2) identification of patient health needs which require the expertise of the pharmacist, (3) development of a program to train patients in the drug therapy program, (4) presentation of a written proposal for review by the hospital administration, (5) presentation of the proposal to third-party representatives, (6) development of accounting procedures to begin charging for clinical services, and (7) provision of a follow-up report to third-party providers on the program's progress. The procedures and problems associated with each step are detailed. The hospitalization cost savings of the program are discussed.

References, 6. *Key words:* Inpatient settings.

NOLD, EDWARD G.; and PATHAK, DEV S. *American Journal of Hospital Pharmacy* 34 (8):823–826, August 1977.

The Uniform Cost Accounting Approach for Pharmacy Pricing Decisions

215 The Uniform Cost Accounting System (UCAS) is an approach designed to improve the procedures used to document the true economic costs involved in providing pharmaceutical services in the community pharmacy. The features and goals of its various accounting components are discussed. An application of the system is described. Four alternative approaches to establishing an equitable reimbursement fee for pharmacists are discussed: (1) administrative fiat, without input from the pharmacist, (2) "jawboning" between program administrators and pharmacists, (3) legal remedies by either party, and (4) periodic (ad hoc) surveys of pharmacy operating data. The need for the UCAS because of current and proposed Medicaid controls (e.g., Maximum Allowable Cost) is discussed.

References, 23. *Key words:* Maximum allowable cost.

SIECKER, BRUCE R. *Journal of the American Pharmaceutical Association NS17* (4):208–212, April 1977.

1976

Comprehensive Pharmacy Cost-Finding. The Path to Pharmacist Satisfaction

213 The pressure of third-party payers for economic accountability has found pharmacists unable to comprehensively document dispensing costs. Factors which have historically hindered a holistic approach to pharmacy cost-finding are: the relegation of accounting to a secondary consideration in pharmacist training; major inadequacies in system purpose in pharmacy accounting; single-entry recordation subsuming the prescription department into the drugstore as a whole; and developmental variance, with many "cigar-box" pharmacies alongside a few that use sophisticated recording and cost-accounting principles. Approaches to prescription pricing have included: use of tradition—analogous to "usual and customary" charges—with year-end evaluation of profit and loss; market interpretation, with the pharmacist charging whatever the local market will bear and assuming part of the drugstore net profit reflects prescriptions; drug program reimbursement formulas, single price offerings based on "gut feel" or what others are doing, in which fees have remained static while costs escalated; periodic surveys assuming a totally nonexistent uniform validity of information.

A clearly superior approach—though it is a long-range project—is the Uniform Cost Accounting System (UCAS), based on redesigning the accounting function to produce needed cost information as a direct output. Its four major characteristics are: uniform recording and interpretation; comprehensive cost documentation; segmentation of the income statement to identify the economic parameters of the prescription department automatically; and two-dimensional cost assignment, with direct costs assigned to appropriate operating departments and residual or unidentified costs to one or more cost centers that are then allocated to the operating departments. Present research being undertaken in Ohio and California on system compatibility and operation is phase one of a three-part developmental pathway. The final version should be tested at a regional or, preferably, at a national level with government underwriting. Finally, a large-scale checkout would help minimize any scale-up problems.

References, 0.

SIECKER, BRUCE R. *California Pharmacist* 24 (*1*):18–19, July 1976.

A Multi-Site Implementation and Evaluation of the Uniform Cost Accounting System for Pharmacy

214

The purpose of a uniform cost accounting system (UCAS) for pharmacy operations is to provide a "comprehensive method for recording and reporting the true economic cost of providing pharmaceutical services." Ten Ohio pharmacies and six California pharmacies volunteered to participate in a study to evaluate the proposed accounting procedures. The pharmacies selected differed in terms of length of operation, type, location and organizational form, and they all dealt with several third-party drug programs. Operating manuals and recording forms were prepared and tailored as necessary to fit the individual pharmacy. The system includes double entry bookkeeping, an accrual basis for recording revenues and expenses, and economic segmentation of the prescription department from the rest of the pharmacy. Pharmacists need to be persuaded of the benefits of a proper accounting system; they tend to under-report their true costs. Specific details and forms for the UCAS treatment of revenues and expenses are included.

References, 64, *Tables,* 16.

SIECKER, BRUCE R. Washington, D.C., American Pharmaceutical Association Foundation, 1976.

On Measuring the Effect of State Reimbursement Policy on Medicaid Spending for Prescription Drugs

246 Cost and quality data from 25 state programs that pay approximately 90 per cent of Medicaid benefits are analyzed to see if the relative efficiency of the programs in delivering prescription drugs can be ascertained. Effects of policy decisions by state legislatures and program officials are explored and interstate comparisons, before and after Medicaid comparisons, and combined comparisons are offered. Adjustments are made for state demographic differences, as well as for differences in prices and available medical services; however, these factors do not explain satisfactorily the state variations in spending for Medicaid services. The author recommends the development of specifications for more efficient and consistent data collection.

In a critique of the study, William G. Shoemaker notes additional problems in making interstate comparisons: differences in eligible populations, in determining eligibility, in medical services and in reported Medicaid spending. Analysts must also consider prescription reimbursement procedures, drug cost determination, the use of formularies, bioequivalency assurance and drug supply. He reviews the generic/brand name controversy and concludes that there is no direct relationship between quality and price of drug products, whether brand name or generic equivalent. He notes that the initiation of a formulary requires a program of physician education. Physicians' prescribing and treatment prerogatives must be protected in order to guarantee high quality medical care. Prescription reimbursement policies must offer incentives. The cost of dispensing a prescription, regardless of the method of payment, should be based on the total cost of the operation of a prescription department.

T. Donald Rucker comments that providers, when faced with inadequate compensation or excessive delay in payment, will find ways to adjust that will increase overall program costs (for example, filing claims for products more expensive than those actually dispensed). He recommends a uniform cost accounting system for all providers and characterizes the Medicaid recordkeeping system as a "national disgrace." He recommends a national commitment to standardization of health care data collection, the training of personnel for computerized information processing, and the coordination of the system to meet the many needs of program planning and administration.

References, not counted; footnotes used. *Key words:* Formularies, substitution.

TRAPNELL, GORDON R. *In* Mitchell, Samuel A.; and Link, Emery A., Editors. *Impact of Public Policy on Drug Innovation and Pricing.* Proceedings of the Third Seminar on Pharmaceutical Public Policy Issues, December 1975. Washington, D.C., American University, 1976. Pages 195–222, 223–230, 230–233.

1975

Economics of Institutional Pharmacy Services under National Health Insurance in Australia

35

The National Health Scheme, which includes a Universal Pharmaceutical Benefits Scheme, was introduced in Australia in the early 1950's. It is estimated that 90 per cent of all outpatient prescription drugs are provided under the Pharmaceutical Benefits Scheme today. Governmental control over drug costs and the provision of pharmacy services are discussed. For each prescription dispensed, all community pharmacists are reimbursed on the basis of a "30 per cent loading on the wholesale price of drugs" in addition to a professional fee, which is negotiated between the Pharmacy Guild and the government. The fee-for-service system helps to ensure that a pharmacist is adequately compensated for increased workloads. Acquisition costs are negotiated between the Australian Minister for Health and the drug manufacturers. The use of a national formulary provides additional control over the drug manufacturers and over the prices for the drugs.

The method of reimbursement of public institutions for the cost of pharmaceutical services under the National Health Scheme is negotiated between the federal Minister for Health and the respective state ministers. The official policy of the federal government is to finance the costs of benefit drugs which are available in community practice; however, in effect, the government reimburses institutions for the costs of all drugs. Figures on the growth in demand for institutional services and the attendant costs of pharmaceutical services are presented. Several shortcomings of the present system of institutional reimbursement are outlined. A recently passed Health Insurance Act included the provision for a cost sharing agreement between the federal and state governments to equally finance hospital expenses, including the cost of pharmaceutical services. While the new system does improve the system of hospital financing, several questions are raised about the methods in which the cost of pharmaceutical services is controlled. The establishment of an Australian Pharmaceutical Commission is proposed and its prospective responsibilities are outlined.

References, 2. *Key words:* Formularies, inpatient settings.

BROOKS, GEOFFREY E.; and KNAPP, DAVID A. *American Journal of Hospital Pharmacy 32 (10)*:1018–1022, October 1975.

Research Report. Allocation of Pharmacist Time for Third Party Prescription Plans

53

Pharmacist time devoted to clerical and other duties necessitated by third-party prescriptions was observed in 20 pharmacies of an eastern metropolitan area chain. With the number of persons covered by private health insurance plans for out-of-hospital prescribed drugs steadily increasing, the demands made on pharmacists for processing third-party claims require investigation. A random sample of 20 pharmacies was selected and observations made of pharmacist activity at three-minute intervals for 36 hours in each pharmacy, a total of 14,400 observations of 93 pharmacists.

Twenty-eight classes of activity were observed, three of which related exclusively to third-party prescriptions: (1) clerical (recordkeeping or processing tasks); (2) communication with patients (explaining drug coverage, for example); (3) specific information acquisition (for example, obtaining drug codes from a manual). It was found that pharmacists spent 1.61 minutes per hour on third-party activities (mostly on clerical tasks) or 2.12 minutes more per prescription than required by prescriptions paid for directly. These figures do not include possible time spent on third-party prescriptions by pharmacists off the job (reading claims information at home, for example) or by nonprofessional staff.

Pharmacist time devoted to third-party activities may be influenced by (1) prescription volume and (2) size and level of staff in the prescription department. Data supported the hypothesis that increased prescription volume would increase the amount of third-party activity. However, contrary to expectations, increases in nonprofessional personnel significantly increased the time devoted to third-party activities, and staff pharmacists spent significantly more time on third-party activities than did manager pharmacists. The authors suggest additional research to determine the feasibility of transferring some third-party prescription activities to nonprofessional staff, and to encourage third-party plan administrators to consider how their claims regulations affect pharmacist activities.

References, 13.

DICKSON, W. MICHAEL; and RODOWSKAS, CHRISTOPHER A., JR. *Inquiry 12* (3):263–267, September 1975.

Community Pharmacy. Pharmacy and the National Health Service. Contractors' Attitudes

114

A 1972 survey of chemist contractors revealed general dissatisfaction with National Health Service (NHS) contract remuneration, but little understanding of the philosophy behind it. Questionnaires were sent to 1465 pharmacy owners concerning their satisfaction with contract remuneration and terms of service. There were 821 representative usable responses.

Over 74 per cent were "dissatisfied" or "very dissatisfied" with remuneration, and 41.3 per cent were unhappy with nonfinancial aspects. The most frequent comment concerned inadequate remuneration, particularly too low "on cost." The second most frequent criticism concerned ingredient cost reimbursement, particularly the level of automatic discounts. Other complaints included the reimbursement of pharmacists compared to other groups, rota and out-of-hours payments, lag behind inflation and return on capital. Contrary to expectation, contractors in large pharmacies were just as dissatisfied. Some contractors actually admitted ignorance about other terms of service. The biggest complaint was long hours. A number thought the total system was too inflexible and would have liked, for example, more leeway for professional judgment and initiative in providing service. Mistrust of the pricing bureau doubtless stems from a faulty understanding of Drug Tariff procedures.

A more legitimate grievance is the requirement for a prescriber counter-signature on prescriptions that are clarified when dispensed. Other concerns were professional status, rota service organization, etc. Even allowing for the limitations of a postal survey, confusion and misconceptions about the contract were apparent in the comments made (and also reflected in the Linstead report). Few contractors saw remuneration as the composite yield of on-cost and professional fee. Revisions since 1972 may have assuaged some dissatisfaction. However, most contractors seem not to be aware that the "improvements" in distribution may represent a gain for some at the expense of others. Part of the problem is the system's complexity, but the Central NHS Committee definitely must upgrade education and the contractors' new association (Counterbalance), for improved communication certainly warrants support.

References, 23.

JONES, I.F. *The Pharmaceutical Journal 215* (5831):150–153, August 16, 1975.

Community Pharmacy. Pharmacy and the National Health Service. A Proposed New Charter for Pharmacy

115

Following a brief review of the philosophy of, and practical problems associated with, current remuneration practices, a "charter" is proposed to solve the imbalance in the current system of remuneration for the pharmacist under the British National Health Service (NHS).

The proposed method of remuneration would not be based on the number of prescriptions dispensed. Six "allocation" elements of NHS remuneration are suggested and discussed: (1) basic practice allowance, (2) seniority payments, (3) retirement benefit, (4) practice relocation fee to encourage equal distribution of pharmacists, (5) fee for late night and emergency dispensing services, and (6) holiday and vacation fees. Fifteen advantages of the reallocation scheme are detailed, for example: (1) removal of the profit from the provision of the pharmaceutical service, (2) provision of a guaranteed income, (3) provision of a career structure for community pharmacists through the seniority payment component, and (4) provision for increased and more realistic planning of the NHS pharmaceutical service. Conditions which would need to be fulfilled by the pharmacist and the pharmacy are outlined. Several potential problems are raised, for example: (1) the difficulty in fairly distributing the workload, (2) the system might necessitate the registration of patients with a particular pharmacy, and (3) that of capital investment and the ownership of property, stock and fixtures.

References, 22.

JONES, I.F. *The Pharmaceutical Journal 215* (5834):211–214, September 6, 1975.

Pharmacy and the National Health Service 1. Some Basic Issues

116 Provisions of the National Insurance Act of 1911, the forerunner of the current National Health Services (NHS) Act, are detailed in order to provide a historical and philosophical background to contract remuneration for chemist contractors under the NHS. Beginning in 1916, payments were made on a "cost price" tariff, in which the contractor received the estimated cost price for the drugs dispensed plus a specified remuneration per prescription for professional services and overhead. This system has caused considerable frustration among chemists during its 60-year history. Many of the same basic issues have been raised over the years: who should negotiate for the contractors? should threatened stoppage of services be used in bargaining? and should the number of pharmacies or NHS contracts be limited by statute?

The chemists have historically bargained from a weak and disunited position and have reacted to external factors rather than controlled them. Historically, there has been no clear basis on which prescription remuneration has been founded. The dependence of pharmacies on NHS contracts for financial success has increased from 6 per cent in the late 1940's to 50 per cent in 1974. The decline in the number of pharmacies throughout the years is a trend which is expected to continue, and which will pose problems for the public, the profession and the State.

References, 34.

JONES, I.F.; and BOOTH, T.G. *The Pharmaceutical Journal 215* (5828):72–74, July 26, 1975.

Pharmacy and the National Health Service 2. Macro-Economic Aspects and Trends

117 Problems and issues associated with the remuneration system of the National Health Service (NHS), in which chemist contractors are paid on an item of service basis, are discussed. The number of prescriptions dispensed determines the amount of payment received with this system of remuneration. Since 1949, prescriptions have increased in number by 46 per cent and in total cost by 900 per cent, most of which is due to higher costs. Various cost figures (e.g., total cost per item, gross margin) are given for each year from 1949–74. In real terms, the average on-cost plus professional fee increased only 10.7 per cent from 1949 to 1975. In real terms, a typical pharmacy owner received in 1974 approximately twice the gross profit per pharmacy received in 1949. This increase is due to a 46 per cent increase in the number of prescriptions dispensed and a 20 per cent decline in the number of pharmacies and is not due to a greater unitary payment rate. For the same reason, the average total net profit per pharmacy (1964–70) has kept pace with the cost-of-living index. Chemist contractors have received a declining portion of NHS expenditures from 1953–72.

The number of prescriptions dispensed is analyzed by pharmacy size classification; in the future, it is expected that half of the pharmacies in England and Wales will be dispensing 75 per cent of the total number of prescriptions. The remaining 50 per cent of the pharmacies will be predominantly independently owned pharmacies located primarily in local communities.

References, 21.

JONES, I.F.; and BOOTH, T.G. *The Pharmaceutical Journal 215* (5829):96–99, August 2, 1975.

Nursing Home Care in the United States: Failure in Public Policy

249

This paper analyzes drug distribution in 23,000 United States nursing homes (1959–1974) and gives examples and testimony supporting lax controls and the unfortunate consequences for both the nursing home patient and the American taxpayer.

Drug distribution in nursing homes is inefficient and ineffective. Physicians are rarely in attendance and nurses are overworked, so too often the responsibility for administering medication falls to aides and orderlies who have had little training. Nursing homes are the most likely places for adverse drug reactions and 20–40 per cent of drugs administered are in error. Patients are frequently tranquilized to keep them quiet; tranquilizers constitute almost 20 per cent of all drugs administered in nursing homes. Kickbacks from the pharmacy to the nursing home operator for the privilege of filling nursing home prescriptions amount to approximately 25 per cent of total prescription charges. This is aggravated when public reimbursement programs such as Medicaid/Medicare allow the nursing home to act as a "middle man" between the pharmacy and the source of payment. Public Law 92-603 (November 1972) prohibits kickbacks, but HEW has never published regulations to implement or enforce the law. Periodic medical review of long-term care facilities and treatment is recommended.

References, 0.

UNITED STATES SENATE. SPECIAL COMMITTEE ON AGING. Subcommittee on Long-Term Care. Supporting Paper No. 2: *Drugs in Nursing Homes: Misuse, High Costs, and Kickbacks.* Ninety-fourth Congress. First Session. Washington D.C., United States Government Printing Office, 1975.

1974

Communications

65

Fletcher's comments are a reply to a 1972 article by Gagnon and Rodowskas, which in turn is followed by a counter-reply by Gagnon and Rodowskas. The two problems discussed are the disagreement between pharmacists and third-party carriers over the definition and methods of determining: (1) prescription ingredient cost, and (2) professional service reimbursement. Fletcher asserts that the difficulty in determining actual prescription ingredient and professional service costs is due to a "philosophical" disagreement between pharmacists and third-party carriers concerning the profit factor included in prescription drug charges submitted for reimbursement.

Gagnon and Rodowskas counter with the argument that the difficulty lies in "technical obstacles," e.g., problems in cost allocation of overhead (e.g., electricity) in an outpatient pharmacy. The "fixed professional fee" and the "usual and customary charge" concepts for determining professional service reimbursement are reviewed, with different interpretations, in each commentary.

Fletcher concludes that the logical solution to the problems between third-party carriers and pharmacists with respect to cost factors underlying the reimbursement schedule, is for the carrier to adopt a benefit that provides direct payments on the basis of actual ingredient cost plus a fixed professional fee. The major benefit of the suggested benefit schedule is that third-party carriers would no longer perpetuate the allegedly inequitable pricing system used by retail pharmacists. Gagnon and Rodowskas claim Fletcher's solution would not solve the problem for three reasons, which are discussed in detail. Gagnon and Rodowskas believe that her solution would, in fact, make coverage more expensive due to increased administrative costs.

References, 10.

See abstract 78, page 165.

FLETCHER, LINDA P.; GAGNON, JEAN P.; and RODOWSKAS, CHRISTOPHER A., JR. *The Journal of Risk and Insurance 41* (4):739–747, December 1974.

Reimbursement Methods for Pharmaceutical Service

76

The three methods of third-party reimbursement currently vying for favor—(1) fixed professional fee, (2) variable professional fee, and (3) usual-and-customary charges—are described in terms of two variables: prescription percentage markups and ingredient costs. In both methods (1) and (2), the relationship between variables is clearly inverse, because the same fee is used for expensive and inexpensive prescriptions. The picture in method (3) is more complex, because consumer pressures affect drug pricing relatively slowly and pharmacists, until recent years, usually followed the convenient practice of assigning a uniform percentage markup to ingredient costs.

A study was conducted to test the assumption that pharmacists, even those still claiming to use a fixed markup, actually tend to use minimum charges for low-cost items (presumably to recover service costs and impress patients with the low price of prescriptions) and competitively lowered markups for rarer high-cost items. Data on 300 prescriptions were collected from each of 29 pharmacies, which represented a mixture of sizes, prescription volumes, service levels, and types, in a six-county region centered on a major urban community. Data included quantity dispensed and price per prescription, cost of stock bottles, quantities in bottles, dosage form, drug type, whether invoice cost was on packages, pharmacists' statement of pricing method, wholesaler's average monthly discount and, for chain pharmacies, warehouse costs and annual direct discounts.

A regression analysis yielded a significant negative correlation (coefficient r^2) between ingredient costs and the computer-calculated markup percentages. A three-dimensional analogue model of the distributions indicated that markup percentages did tend to decline as cost increased, most prescriptions had costs below $3, and some had low markup percentages. Plotting of each pharmacy's markups showed a nonuniform but down-sloping relationship between variables. Prescriptions with the same ingredient costs often had different markups, probably because different turnover indicators, e.g., dosage form or drug category, were being considered in pricing.

References, 6.

GAGNON, JEAN P.; and RODOWSKAS, CHRISTOPHER A., JR. *Journal of the American Pharmaceutical Association NS14* (*12*):675–678, December 1974.

A Study of the Relationships of Drug Dosage Form, Therapeutic Class and Pharmaceutical Services with the Gross Margins on Prescription Drugs

77

Retail prescription prices depend on overhead and professional expenses, variables such as drug dosage form (tablet or capsule, liquid, ointment, suppository, eye-ear-nose preparation, injectable), therapeutic class (maintenance or nonmaintenance) and level of pharmaceutical service (delivery, patient record card and accounts receivable services, with 3 gradations noted of each of these services). The latter 3 variables were correlated with prescription ingredient cost for 300 new prescriptions from each of 29 pharmacies in a three-county area and the gross margins were calculated. Markup data for dosage forms and therapeutic classes were treated by analysis of variance and covariance; levels of service were analyzed by regression methods. Markup data collected from the pharmacies included quantity dispensed, price per prescription, quantity and cost of stock bottles, dosage form, type of drug, companies with which direct accounts were maintained, and levels of service. Wholesalers supplied data on average monthly purchases and wholesale discounts. Chain pharmacies supplied warehouse costs and annual direct discounts.

Significant differences ($p = 0.05$) were found with dosage form, therefore dosage form may affect prescription dollar and percentage markups. No significant differences exist for dollar or percentage markups between maintenance and nonmaintenance drugs when prescription ingredient costs are controlled. Prescription ingredient costs appear to explain the higher dollar markups for maintenance drugs. However, most maintenance drugs are for larger quantities and therefore prescriptions last longer and are refilled less frequently. This should compensate for the effects of high maintenance prescription prices on low-income patients (especially people over 60, the major users of maintenance drugs.) Maintaining family record cards and accounts receivable services (credit cards were accepted by 75 per cent of the pharmacies) did not significantly account for markup variations, but delivery services did contribute significantly to prescription markup percentages.

References, 23.

GAGNON, JEAN P.; and RODOWSKAS, CHRISTOPHER A., JR. *Medical Care 12* (*1*):49–61, January 1974.

National Health Service. Cost of Dispensing in the Pharmaceutical Services

170 The purpose of the study was to determine how much of the cost of the pharmaceutical services of the British National Health Service (NHS) is due to the actual, i.e., manufacturer's, price of drugs. The pharmaceutical contractors are paid by the regional executive council on a standard fee-for-services basis, while the pharmaceutical services of NHS hospitals negotiate drug prices more directly with the drug manufacturers.

Prescription price data were obtained from the Birmingham Pricing Bureau in December, 1972, and were expressed per unit medical manpower (i.e., prescriber). Analysis of prescription price data showed that the NHS hospital price was only 60 per cent of the average payment made to the pharmaceutical contractors if the latter amount included the pharmacist's professional fee, and 80 per cent if it did not. This difference, on the basis of the 60 per cent calculation, would amount to approximately 80 million (English) pounds annually (1972), of which 30 million (English) pounds would represent the difference in drug pricing and 50 million (English) pounds of the cost difference would represent the professional fee and running costs of the pharmaceutical service contractor. The difference in drug pricing results from the hospital practices of bulk purchasing of drugs and of purchasing by generic name. The running costs incurred by the pharmaceutical services contractor and not by the NHS hospital pharmaceutical services include the costs of providing drug quality control testing, maintaining a larger drug inventory and remaining open for business for more hours.

In order to reduce the nationwide costs of pharmaceutical services, an alternative approach to dispensing drugs is suggested. The proposed system would include direct NHS-financed dispensaries attached to existing hospital outpatient departments or to a group practice center with six or more family practitioners. Estimates of cost savings under the proposed system are presented.

References, 6. *Key words:* Direct provision.

OPIT, L.J.; and FARMER, R.D.T. *The Lancet: 1* (7849):160, 162, February 2, 1974.

Public Policy Considerations in the Pricing of Prescription Drugs in the United States

198 The United States spent about $10 billion for prescribed drugs in 1973, and government insurance programs paid over 27 per cent of this amount. Other justifications for government interest in drug pricing are the consumer's relative subservience to his illness, the pharmaceutical marketplace and professional expertise; the presumed high social utility of federal legend products; and the responsibility increasingly delegated to third-party insurers. There are several inadequately discussed problems in the relationship of product pricing to actual cost. Data obtained in 1969 for 9 important pharmaceuticals, which are probably still roughly valid, show that a median of only 9 per cent of wholesale prices represented direct expenses. Standard trade costs from the *Red Book* indicate that active ingredient amounts frequently do not correlate with prices. The relationship between size of package and price is similarly unpredictable.

Another questionable practice is differentiation in price by type of buyer without regard to quantities purchased. The biggest dispensing price problem is how to relate prescription charges to true overhead costs. Studies in several states show a very haphazard relationship now. A uniform cost-accounting system is the obvious solution. Other issues to be settled are an appropriate level of profit, for which a good cost-accounting system is prerequisite, and the role of incentives when both legitimate commercial and professional interests are involved.

Problems with prescription price posting—its promotional aspects, relative lack of effect on product cost and operational defects—can be minimized by adoption of a 1972 California Pharmaceutical Association proposal that pharmacies simply post a flat overhead fee to be applied to all prescriptions. Listing the dispensing services involved would further enhance consumer understanding. Third-party programs play a major role in obscuring economic relationships that should be reflected in prescription prices by reimbursing without regard to actual operating expenses or level of professional services. Failure to rationalize pricing mechanisms before a national health insurance program would bring imposed solutions.

References, 5.

RUCKER, T. DONALD. *International Journal of Health Services* 4 (*1*):171–179, Winter 1974.

Professional and Economic Bases for Pharmaceutical Services under the British National Health Service

227

The British National Health Service (NHS) system for reimbursing pharmacy owners is described. A committee of pharmacy representatives negotiates with the government for remuneration, to include: (1) container cost, negotiated after a cost survey, (2) ingredient cost, based on manufacturer or wholesale price, (3) overhead costs, based on a dispensing costs inquiry every few years in sample pharmacies that use work-sampling analyses and financial records to compute a cost per prescription that is updated annually according to certain indices, (4) labor costs, based on data from the work-sampling study, 6 staff categories and a negotiated proprietor's payment that considers hours worked, experience, etc., and (5) profit, a negotiated return on capital. Rising costs have been a serious concern since the 1950's. Data are presented which show changes in remuneration since 1948.

Administrative controls, not stringent by some United States standards, exert pressures toward "rational prescribing." A free *Prescriber's Journal* provides physicians with up-to-date information on drugs; a committee has been formed to evaluate drug effectiveness; NHS annually sends each physician a month's comparison of his prescription quantities with national and local ones and contacts him if there is a large deviation. Placing the main burden for controlling drug utilization on physicians is possible because patients generally see only a single general practitioner or group practice and no refill prescriptions are given.

Patient copayment for prescription drugs, introduced amidst great controversy (and with many exemptions) as a government economy measure, has also moderated demand. Pharmacy owners may receive other compensation, including rural subsidies, rota duty payments for opening outside normal hours, "urgent" fees for emergency dispensing, out-of-pocket expenses, broken bulk payments for packages of drugs not normally stocked and fees for private prescriptions. Arguments through the years have centered on NHS reimbursement amounts and computation methods. A current dispute between the Pharmaceutical Society and the report of a Working Party representing several pharmacist groups concerns such matters as whether the remuneration system is too complicated and whether pharmacist advisory services can be isolated as a cost. General career discontent may be expressing itself in economic grievances.

References, 23. *Key words:* Drug utilization review, patient cost sharing.

SMITH, MICKEY C.; JONES, IAN; and BOOTH, T. GEOFFREY. *Drugs in Health Care 1* (2):59–73, Fall 1974.

1973

The Capitation System for Pharmaceutical Services

181 A new concept in the payment for pharmaceutical services has been suggested, the capitation system, which would eliminate the incentive for the pharmacist to dispense higher-cost drugs. Traditionally, pharmacist reimbursement has been based on the drug prescribed, through the percentage markup system. Preferable to that, however, has been the professional fee system, where a flat amount is added to the cost of the product, thereby distributing more equitably the cost of services. While this is more reflective of actual costs and proves to be more equitable to the patron, most pharmacists have continued using the markup system. With the proposed alternative, the pharmacist would charge for drugs at cost and the patron would be encouraged to patronize the same establishment. Furthermore, it would allow for the maintenance of complete patron medication records. While this concept has been implemented only minimally, it seems ideal for institutional (i.e., hospital) settings, where patients would pay for drugs at cost and according to usage, as well as a daily flat rate for drug-related services. The conclusion is that whatever method of remuneration for services is used, the provision of the drugs themselves must be set apart from the reimbursement for them.

References, 3. *Key words:* Direct provision.

PROVOST, GEORGE, P. *American Journal of Hospital Pharmacy 30* (6): 493, June 1973.

Research Report. Paying the Pharmacist under the British National Health Service

228 The administrative mechanism used in England to remunerate pharmacists for their services is thoroughly discussed. The system handled 247 million prescriptions in 1971. The reimbursement situation in England differs from that of the United States in a number of ways, for example: (1) the larger number of prescriptions in the United States would create problems not encountered in Britain and (2) certain United States state and federal regulations, e.g., maintenance of prescriptions on file by the pharmacist, would prohibit the wholesale transfer of prescriptions as now takes place in the current British system. The administrative organization and claims handling operations of the Joint Pricing Committee and the regional pricing bureaux are described in detail. The timing and method of calculation of payment to the pharmacist by his local Executive Council is explained.

The four components of the prescription payment are: (1) net price of drug dispensed, which is determined by negotiation, (2) a professional fee for each prescription, (3) an "on-cost" allowance and (4) a container allowance. The profit for the pharmacist is included in the professional fee and "on-cost" allowance components. Surveys are conducted throughout England and Wales every three years to determine average overhead and labor costs for pharmacists, in order to calculate, respectively, the "on-cost" allowance and the professional fee. The system includes a copayment mechanism, in which a flat amount (20 pence in 1973) per prescription is paid by the patient. About half of all patients are exempted, for a variety of reasons, from the copayment. The copayment mechanism was re-introduced in 1968, after which there was a 7 per cent reduction in the number of prescriptions dispensed in the following twelve-month period. Computers are not used in claims processing, since automation cannot be economically justified due to the low administrative costs of the present system. Utilization review is manually performed, thus limiting the number of innovations which could be introduced to improve its sophistication. Both physicians and pharmacists are checked periodically to guard against prescribing and processing abuses.

References, 20. *Key words:* Drug utilization review, patient cost sharing.

SMITH, MICKEY, C.; JONES, IAN; and BOOTH, T. GEOFFREY. *Inquiry 10* (3):57–64, September 1973.

1972
Prescription Cost Determination in Kansas

47

The methodology for a survey undertaken to objectively determine community pharmacy prescription dispensing costs is described. The Kansas Department of Social Welfare agreed to sponsor the statewide survey and base its Title XIX reimbursements on it. Questionnaires on the previous year were returned by 449 of 627 pharmacies in 1970 and 458 of 645 in 1971. One section asked for information such as net acquisition cost and dispensing charge for the first 50 new prescriptions at two-month intervals; the second requested descriptive and operating characteristics and some 48 items of expense data. Calculations at the University of Kansas school of pharmacy established an average daily number of prescriptions, validated time spent by managers in prescription departments and checked various items for internal and external consistency. Missing items were filled in on the bases of area averages, personal contacts, experience in past surveys, etc.

Pharmacists tended to understate expenses. Edited expenses were computer-processed as either (1) professional time or (2) overhead per prescription order. The printout showed the average charge, cost of goods sold and gross and net profit per prescription by parameters such as area population and annual sales volume. Some findings of interest were marked variations in dispensing costs and the fact that one-fourth of the pharmacies gained little or nothing over expenses on prescriptions (23 pharmacies charged less than the break-even point). The average dispensing cost for the 1970 data was $1.57. Seven per cent of the pharmacies, which were doing 15 per cent of the prescription dollar volume, had a prescription income greater than $500,000 a year. Chain stores composed 12.5 per cent of the sample, but did 19 per cent of the prescription volume. A field audit of 31 vendors in the 1970 survey indicated that the supplied data were highly accurate and that the pharmacists were very accepting of the long questionnaire.

Future survey improvements would include requesting balance sheet data, better bookkeeping on renewed prescriptions by some pharmacies, less time betweeen cost measurement and reimbursement (now 2 years) and systems for rewarding operating efficiency and factoring in the provision of extensive professional services. Factors in the success of the approach were an unusual degree of cooperation among the parties concerned, (perhaps) a low rate of Title XIX reimbursement, and utmost fairness in the uniform evaluation and adjustment of cost figures and protection of confidentiality.

References, 1.

COTTON, HUGH A.; and RUCKER, T. DONALD. *Journal of the American Pharmaceutical Association NS12* (8):412–415, August 1972.

---

61 Opportunities for a Prepaid Pharmacy Foundation

The community foundation approach to providing pharmaceutical services for prepaid group health programs allows pharmacists to retain authority over delivery of services and to undertake contracts with medical care foundations, group practice plans and government agencies. Paralleling the development of foundations for medical care (groups of physicians who maintain independent practice but function as a group with regard to standards and utilization review), local foundations for the practice of pharmacy provide the means by which pharmacists can participate equally in the health care delivery system. (In prepaid group plans such as Kaiser-Permanente, pharmacists are employees with little responsibility for the administration or control of pharmaceutical services.)

Medical care foundations are equipped to negotiate and administer prepaid health care programs. This has been studied in the Medi-Cal (California) contract with the San Joaquin Foundation for Medical Care. The Foundation provides physician and pharmaceutical services to eligible recipients in the area. The state makes prospective monthly payments based on the number of eligible persons and category of assistance and also reimburses the Foundation for administrative costs. The physician is rewarded for providing only those services which are essential; this requires enforceable standards and peer review to insure quality of health care.

The Foundation project saves California 10 per cent over the previous cost of delivering Medi-Cal services. The pharmaceutical service saves 10–15 per cent, due to a drug utilization review program administered by the PAID Prescriptions organization and the San Joaquin County Pharmaceutical Society.

The California Pharmaceutical Association (CPhA) is developing a state foundation for pharmaceutical services which will negotiate and administer prepaid contracts for the provision of pharmaceutical services through local pharmacies. The CPhA will encourage local pharmaceutical associations to form foundations to set standards for services, including record-keeping practices, the establishment of a formulary and the participation in local area health education programs, as well as claims processing, utilization review and the maintenance of drug profiles. Peer and drug utilization review programs (on both over and underutilization of drugs) must be interdisciplinary for maximum effectiveness. The foundation approach will allow local pharmaceutical foundations to participate with local medical care foundations in providing an integrated program of health services in a geographic area on a prepaid contract basis.

References, 2. *Key words:* Drug utilization review.

FINCH, DENNIS K. *Journal of the American Pharmaceutical Association* NS12 (4):173–175, April 1972.

Two Controversial Problems in Third Party Outpatient Prescription Plans

78

In the mid sixties, insurance experts were predicting that outpatient prescription drug coverage would expand rapidly in the years to come. By 1970, however, only 15 per cent of outpatient prescription charges were paid for by third parties. The authors ascribe this slow growth to difficulties in four major areas: (1) the large number of small claims generated by drug coverage, (2) the high cost of processing each claim, (3) the high risk to insurance companies because of the widespread utilization of drugs, and (4) difficulties associated with reimbursing pharmacists for product cost and dispensing services. This article focuses specifically on the fourth problem area.

A brief chronology of the growth of private and public drug insurance is presented, followed by a more detailed analysis of the ingredient cost controversy and the professional fee controversy.

The major problem in determining ingredient cost is that different pharmacies pay different prices for drug products. Insurance companies and government programs took the position that they would reimburse the actual acquisition cost. Pharmacists, on the other hand, argue for reimbursement based on average wholesale costs, which were estimated to be 10–15 per cent higher than actual acquisition costs. The authors suggest that a uniform cost for prescription drugs be set that is halfway between average wholesale and actual acquisition costs.

Insurance companies wish to avoid reimbursing for professional services on the basis of usual and customary charges because of auditing difficulties and the ease with which such charges may rise. Most plans chose to reimburse pharmacists on the basis of a fixed professional fee. These programs ran into legal difficulties in the 1960's however. In 1969, the Virginia Supreme Court ruled that the use of a fixed fee by Blue Cross was a "per se" violation of price fixing. Soon thereafter, the Illinois Supreme Court ruled the opposite in a similar case. Government programs are not bound by these decisions and the Medicaid program favors a fixed fee for reimbursement.

References, 18.

See abstract 65, page 157.

GAGNON, JEAN P.; and RODOWSKAS, CHRISTOPHER A., Jr. *Journal of Risk and Insurance* 39 (4):603–611, December 1972.

1971

Statement

85

The retail pharmacy is bearing the burden of an unjust method of reimbursement from third-party plans. In a 1970 study of about 2000 pharmacies nationwide, R. A. Gosselin & Company show that 89 per cent of pharmacists are unhappy with an inflexible fixed fee-for-service method. This system ignores the factors, e.g., geographic, socio-economic, services rendered by pharmacists, purchasing service, etc., that affect operating costs among pharmacies. As these elements change, the price for a prescription will vary, even from a single pharmacy, over a given period of time. The method of averaging provides an inequitable system for practically everyone, with half the pharmacies operating at a loss while the other half make an excessive profit. A sample covering eleven states shows that these many factors can cause a deviation in cost for prescription services ranging from +27.2 to −25.9. Displeasure is voiced by 67 per cent of the pharmacists surveyed regarding the waiting period for payment. Only 19 per cent of pharmacies routinely receive payment within 30 days, while roughly one-third do not receive payment for up to two months after the prescription is dispensed. Three per cent experienced a delay of payment of greater than four months. The only equitable fee system is one that reflects the variables pertaining to each pharmacy. This individualized method would determine each fee based on historical and current experience of that pharmacy.

References, 0.

GOSSELIN, RAYMOND. In United States House of Representatives. Hearings before the Subcommittee on Environmental Problems Affecting Small Business of the Select Committee on Small Business. *Third-Party Prepaid Prescription Programs.* Ninety-second Congress. First Session. Washington, D.C., United States Government Printing Office, 1971. Pages 154–162.

Pharmacy Charges for Prescription Drugs under Third Party Programs. Variability Analysis

86

This report is a summary of the results of a comprehensive statistical analysis of variability in nearly half a million prescription charges and the operating characteristics of more than 2600 United States retail pharmacies. The analysis was jointly commissioned by the National Association of Retail Druggists and the National Association of Chain Drug Stores to aid third-party reimbursement administrators and planners in establishing equitable reimbursement policies. (A 402-page technical report submitted in January 1971 presents the complete findings.) The report discusses the objectives, methodology and major findings of the study, problems with present reimbursement methods (determining product and dispensing costs), problems with claims processing (submission procedures and waiting period for payment) and the Prescription Services Index (PSI) prediction model as a workable reimbursement alternative to a fixed or variable dispensing fee plus cost. The calculated PSI considers regional differences, urbanization and variable income levels, store characteristics, third-party prescription involvement, customer services, sources of drugs, personnel, community relations and professional development.

References, 0.

GOSSELIN, R.A. AND COMPANY. Final Report. Dedham, Massachusetts, R.A. Gosselin and Company, 1971.

Review Article. Paying for Outpatient Prescription Drugs and Related Services in Third Party Programs

128

Rapidly expanding third-party drug coverage warrants review of reimbursement mechanisms. Some $4 billion was spent on outpatient prescription drugs in 1970. Independent pharmacies represent 80 per cent of the outlets, but "corporate" pharmacies are increasing and now sell almost one-third of the prescriptions. The present salary structure tends to ignore quality of service. Prescription pricing often bears little relationship to costs because of the many variables in drug distribution and the difficulties of allocating overhead expenses. The majority of pharmacists now add a sliding percentage markup to different drug cost ranges. Some writers advocate adding a professional fee to drug costs. Which method is more fair is arguable. Most pharmacists use personally developed methods, leading to well documented price variability.

The design of a reimbursement plan involves program characteristics (eligibility, scope of benefits, administration, etc.) plus specific drug component attributes. These include the high potential for increase in drug utilization under a prepayment plan implied by comparative studies; the relatively easily expanded drug supply and commercial drug promotion; the unique combination of product and service components; and the low average claim size with a potential for very many claims. Third parties may provide drug services directly or reimburse either the client or the vendor. Combination programs are unduly complicated. Reimbursement can exert more control in the more popular vendor programs, with client copayments used to offset the costs of higher utilization and claim submission in this system.

Existing programs reveal a variety of ways to determine the amount of reimbursements. The Task Force on Prescription Drugs' criteria for a good system include payment based on costs, with rewards for efficient use of resources, holding down costs of drug therapy, simplicity, promotion of high quality drugs and services and reasonable administrative costs. Rucker adds that it should be responsive to cost fluctuations, not favor a particular type of outlet, and reflect true differences in costs and services. Reimbursement of usual and customary charges is used in many client payment programs and some vendor plans. It offers least pharmacist resistance but is difficult to audit. A 1970 drugstore-commissioned study proposed using various factors to set a maximum for reimbursement, but the plan has obvious flaws. Prepaid group practice capitation payment systems are simpler because most groups operate their own pharmacies, but most independent pharmacies could not undertake this. Separating reimbursement formulas for drugs and dispensing services offers greater flexibility and control. One base used for drug cost is actual acquisition cost. Critics cite a lack of provision for costs of obtaining purchase discounts, potential encouragement of deceptive distribution practices and difficulties in developing satisfactory audit procedures.

More popular, and probably more satisfactory, is the use of a variant of standard cost—simple use of an available price book to set standard wholesale cost, or setting a maximum allowable cost on multiple-source products, which achieves savings only with generic prescribing. Some way to reward efficient purchasing and lower program costs must be found. Surveys show third parties also use very diverse methods to reimburse for dispensing costs. Most formulas are based on either percentage markups or flat fees. The General Accounting Office charges that markups encourage the dispensing of expensive products when possible. Fixed fees are often perceived by pharmacists as too low and generally have little relation to costs. There are also legal questions involved. Antitrust laws have been applied against pharmacists meeting to discuss fees. The status of third-party fee setting is still unclear. Published surveys can be a rough guide to fee levels. Several formulas have been proposed to determine costs in individual pharmacies. Most tend to inflate costs. Incentives for improved services have had little attention. A variable fee could be used to stimulate delivery, emergency service, record maintenance, increased dispensing efficiency and pharmacist-patient prescription consultation. A solid cost-based variable fee method for dispensing costs would come closest to meeting the criteria for a good reimbursement system. Current research may yield simpler ways of determining individual dispensing costs. A way must also be found to legally permit greater pharmacist participation.

References, 81. *Key words:* Patient cost sharing.

KNAPP, DAVID, A. *Medical Care Review 28* (8):826–859, August 1971.

Medicaid. Payment of Reasonable Charges for Prescribed Drugs

230

This federally-prepared manual deals with reasonable charges for prescribed drugs and covers the following items: authorization (the law, regulations and other factors); prescription pricing methods and options; variations in reimbursement for prescribed drugs by different types of licensed authorized practitioners; formularies and implementation guidelines.

The federal drug formulary policy states: "The use of a formulary is optional, as are provisions for the use of generic drugs. Where either is employed, there must be standards for quality, safety and effectiveness under the supervision of professional personnel." States implementing formularies should consider these guidelines: medications should meet FDA standards for identity, strength, safety, quality, purity and effectiveness; state agencies should strive for economy consistent with these standards; formularies should be flexible and consider professional prerogatives, formulary committees should include physicians, pharmacologists, pharmacists and other professional personnel to revise the formulary periodically; procedures for additions and deletions to the formulary and for the reimbursement of nonlisted items should be formulated; a code number from the FDA National Drug Code Directory should be assigned to each item for ease of electronic data processing. Hospital formularies offer up-to-date information on drugs and drug therapy and are maintained by a staff committee.

The American Society of Hospital Pharmacists' *American Hospital Formulary Service* distributes guidelines for hospitals to use in preparing their formularies. Approximately 20 states in the Medicaid program control drug costs and prescribing standards through the use of a formulary. Some also limit prescribing to generic drugs and establish a price ceiling. Few states can afford a comprehensive drug service and usually limit reimbursable drugs to those in a formulary. Some states without formularies exclude classes of drugs such as multivitamins. Drugs may have chemical and proprietary names in addition to generic names; dispensing combination products which contain therapeutic equivalents of substances prescribed by generic name can be difficult. The successful formulary in Pennsylvania includes 90 per cent of all commonly used drugs and includes price information on which pharmacists base their markup. In sum, formularies define payable drugs, simplify prescription auditing and processing, as well as drug and price coding, and allow some control over drug prices. However, many physicians will ignore a formulary or see it as interference with professional prerogatives, and formularies may easily become inflexible or outdated.

Appendices present excerpts from Title XIX of the Social Security Act and the *Code of Federal Regulations,* and the Kansas state survey for determination of variable dispensing fees.

References, 0.

SOCIAL AND REHABILITATION SERVICE. MEDICAL SERVICES ADMINISTRATION. DHEW Publication No. SRS-MSA-196-1971. Washington, D.C., United States Government Printing Office, 1971.

Third Party Prepaid Prescription Programs

248

Hearings were held to investigate third-party prepaid prescription programs and their impact on the 40,000 United States independently-owned retail pharmacies. The report includes testimony of pharmacists and pharmacy owners, representatives of professional associations and trade organizations, spokesmen for insurance companies, and officials of the Department of Justice and the Federal Trade Commission. It contains third-party program guidelines, claims and reimbursement forms, letters and reports from other interested parties.

References, 0.

UNITED STATES HOUSE OF REPRESENTATIVES. Hearings before the Subcommittee on Environmental Problems Affecting Small Business of the Select Committee on Small Business. Ninety-second Congress. First Session. Washington, D.C., United States Government Printing Office, 1971.

1970

Problems Facing Pharmacists under Medicare and Medicaid

17

Dr. William S. Apple outlines problems regarding payment for services provided under Medicare and Medicaid and offers possible solutions for these problems. The pharmacist's role in the task of drug use review is discussed at length. This article is a reprint of a statement of the American Pharmaceutical Association to the Subcommittee on Medicare and Medicaid of the Senate Committee on Finance, June 16, 1970.

Problems confronting the pharmacist under Medicare and Medicaid are classified into four areas: (1) inability to obtain prompt reimbursement from fiscal intermediaries, (2) inability to collect from institutional providers of health care who contracted for pharmaceutical services, e.g., nursing homes, (3) ethical and legal problems in the area of kickbacks to health care facilities, a practice deemed necessary in order to obtain contracts for pharmaceutical services and (4) abuses arising out of physician ownership of pharmaceutical facilities.

The problem of the time delay in receiving reimbursement is compounded by the fact that more than 50 per cent of the total claim amount represents reimbursement for the cost of the drug product, which was paid for in advance by the pharmacist. Due to "out-of-pocket" expenses, the pharmacist is often forced to borrow money to meet current operating expenses, a practice which adds to his financial burden since he is not compensated for the cost of borrowing. Pharmacists encounter additional severe difficulties when an across-the-board percentage reduction on the claims of Medicaid providers is imposed by the state. Such a reduction substantially reduces the pharmacist's compensation for his services due to the fixed cost of the drug product.

Two solutions are advanced to solve problems in the area of reimbursement by health care providers: (1) certification by the provider that all suppliers' claims were paid before the provider would receive Medicare and Medicaid funds or (2) direct reimbursement to the supplier by the fiscal intermediary. This latter solution would, in addition, help to remedy the problem of kickback payments by the pharmacist to the health care provider. Since it is impossible to monitor the charges for the 12.5 million prescriptions dispensed annually to extended health care facilities, Dr. Apple proposes that the government require that compensation for pharmaceutical services be based on two components: (1) reimbursement for the cost of the drug and (2) a specified professional fee for the pharmacist's services. A plan employing these two principles devised by the Kansas Pharmaceutical Association and the Kansas Department of Social Welfare is described in detail. Finally, the problems connected with physician ownership of pharmaceutical services are discussed in connection with a Senate bill S.1575, which would prohibit federal financial participation in the cost of drugs under any program in which the medical practitioner has a financial interest in dispensing pharmaceuticals.

The American Pharmaceutical Association's reason for full support of the proposed legislation centers about abuses which occur in such situations and the undermining of the professionalism of pharmacists in situations where a physician controls the selection and dispensing of drugs. The Senate testimony concludes with comments on the pharmacist's role in drug utilization review, his contribution to the assurance of rational drug prescribing and dispensing practices and his contribution as the most knowledgeable source of information on program costs and administrative burdens in third-party programs.

References, 0. *Key words:* Drug utilization review.

APPLE, WILLIAM S. *Journal of the American Pharmaceutical Association NS10* (9): 494–500, September 1970.

Controls over Medicaid Drug Program in Ohio Need Improvement

44

To evaluate the controls established to safeguard Ohio's Medicaid drug program from improper use, the General Accounting Office examined selected case records from the state department of public welfare, two county welfare departments, selected nursing homes and pharmacies, and studied the state policy of paying pharmacies for drugs dispensed, whether prices paid for selected drugs were reasonable, and whether adequate records of drugs administered in nursing homes and dispensed by pharmacies were being kept. Information provided by the state to counties for caseworker determinations of drug usage was reviewed. Agencies were informed of the results of the study.

It was found that certain drugs were not reasonably priced because the state policy of paying pharmacies cost-plus-a-percentage-of-cost gave them an incentive for selling higher-cost drug products. Controls for ensuring that prices billed to the state conformed to state regulations were inadequate. Nursing homes were not obtaining long-term maintenance drugs in economical quantities.

It is recommended that federal assistance be provided to the states in revising their drug payment policies. Guidelines should be issued for drug utilization review, and their implementation should be monitored. Priority should be given to drug efficacy studies on those drug products identified by the HEW Task Force on Prescription Drugs as having the greatest potential for savings; results should be widely disseminated to physicians.

*References,*0. *Key words:* Drug utilization review.

COMPTROLLER GENERAL OF THE UNITED STATES. Washington, D.C., Comptroller General, 1970.

1967

Review of Pricing Methods Used by Various States in the Purchase of Prescribed Drugs under Federally Aided Public Assistance Programs

45

The report reviews prescription drug pricing formulas and prices paid to retail pharmacists for drugs prescribed for welfare recipients (fiscal 1966) under the Social Security Act. Diverse pricing methods were found which, in many states, did not result in equitable prescription drug pricing. A pricing system that includes professional fees should fairly compensate a pharmacy for costs associated with selling, purchasing, direct and indirect cost factors, plus a reasonable allowance for profit. Professional fees were found to range from 50¢ to $1.75, and percentage of cost markups from 50 per cent to $66\frac{2}{3}$ per cent. No justification was found for the great variance among states in amounts allowed pharmacies in excess of the cost of the drug products. The report suggests prohibiting cost-plus-percentage-of-cost pricing methods and recommends cost-plus-fixed-professional-fee basis instead. Flexible professional fees, on a graduated scale with higher fees for higher-cost drugs, may be considered. In 41 states, drugs were provided to welfare recipients through private pharmacies which then billed local or state welfare agencies for payment.

References, 0.

COMPTROLLER GENERAL OF THE UNITED STATES. Report to the United States Congress. Washington, D.C., Comptroller General, 1967.

Cross-References

For further information on reimbursement, see:

ABSTRACT NUMBER	PAGE NUMBER	ABSTRACT NUMBER	PAGE NUMBER
16	34	99	92
18	57	113	41
19	47	120	48
22	41	177	35
24	89	195	21
39	78	212	60
46	18	216	32
56	10	222	77
88	111	240	82
94	23	244	50
97	58	257	62

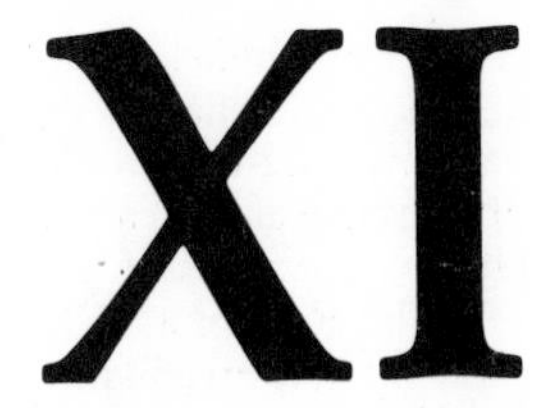

Prescribing Controls: Drug Use Review

Modifying prescribing behavior is the most direct way of affecting the economy and quality of drug use. Drug use review (DUR) is a major approach to producing changes in prescribing. Key words: Drug utilization review.

1977

Drug Usage Screening Criteria

25

Screening criteria for 40 drugs frequently prescribed for adult use (indications for use, minimum/maximum daily dose and length of therapy) and 10 drugs for pediatric use (indications, dose and length of therapy, plus age restrictions) are listed. These criteria may be used to screen large numbers of prescriptions in order to rapidly identify instances of exceptional drug prescribing, which can then be investigated further. Criteria were based on the scientific and professional literature. Combination drugs deemed to be "irrational" were identified, and clinical documentation presented. By indicating that some products fail to meet any criteria for appropriate drug therapy, there is thus an acceptable basis for deciding to exclude these products from a drug list or formulary.

The development of criteria in a drug use review program is not as difficult as getting physicians and pharmacists to accept them. It is useful, therefore, to involve physicians and pharmacists in the development and application of all aspects of a drug use review program.

References 43.

BRANDON, BRENDA M.; KNAPP, DAVID A.; KLEIN, LINDA S.; and GREGORY, JOHN. *American Journal of Hospital Pharmacy* 34 (2):146–151, February 1977.

Model for Drug Usage Review in a Hospital

32

A five-part conceptual model for a hospital drug use review (DUR) program is outlined. The program's components are: (1) authority to operate a DUR program and an authoritative source for decisions regarding resources, procedures and policies; (2) operational characteristics of the delivery system and demographic characteristics of the population served; (3) construction of a baseline drug-use profile; (4) establishment of standards of appropriateness of drug usage; and (5) a plan to evaluate the goals, effectiveness and costs of the DUR. Eight steps of an evaluation program are outlined.

The goals of a DUR program are: (1) improvement in the level of patient care; (2) improvement in the management and use of hospital resources; (3) clarification of the drug component of patient care and better integration of the hospital's pharmaceutical services with other hospital services, and (4) improvement in the "fact-finding capacity" which will help in identifying and solving hospital problems.

References, 4. *Key words:* Inpatient settings.

BRODIE, DONALD C.; SMITH, WILLIAM E.; and HLYNKA, JOHN N. *American Journal of Hospital Pharmacy* 34 (3):251–254, March 1977.

Monitoring Drug Utilization—Modification of Physician Prescribing Habits

119 Physician prescribing problems fall into four categories: treatment failure, iatrogenic diseases, needless risk and economic waste. The occurrence of these problems is widespread. To counter them, it is important to establish a system to collect physician prescribing data, compare them with appropriate standards, institute methods of effecting change and monitor the results.

The prescribing process includes first a diagnosis, followed by the decision as to whether drug therapy is required. If it is, a specific drug must be selected, followed by an appropriate dose, dosage interval and duration of therapy. Each of these decision steps may be the subject of drug use review. Because of the large number of drugs on the market, it would be impractical to attempt to monitor all of them. Fortunately, a relatively small number of drugs accounts for a large number of the prescriptions written. The patient population is also important. Structural difficulties make drug use review on outpatient populations more difficult than on hospitalized patients.

The ideal drug use review system includes a feedback mechanism to help the physician improve prescribing practices. Occasionally, formularies or other restrictive devices have been used to improve prescribing.

In summary, the establishment of a drug use review system is advocated as a potential solution to problems of inappropriate physician prescribing.

References, 4.

KARR, G. *Canadian Journal of Hospital Pharmacy 30* (1):13–15, January-February 1977.

Incorporating Diagnosis Information into a Manual Drug Use Review System

130 In a follow-up to the development of a manual drug use review system based on dispensed outpatient prescription orders, the authors investigated the value of adding diagnosis information to prescriptions to develop more comprehensive and specific screening criteria. They collected data in January-March 1975 from four sites where pharmacists dispensed directly from medical records or prescribers included diagnosis information voluntarily: an urban neighborhood health center, a hospital outpatient pharmacy, a rural ambulatory clinic and an Indian Health Service Hospital outpatient pharmacy. Project staff pharmacists developed criteria for diagnosis and drug match screening to supplement existing criteria for dosage and length of therapy for the 40 most frequently prescribed drugs. After outside review of the criteria, they were applied to collected data and the results computer-processed. Diagnosis was successfully linked with over 90 per cent of 3431 prescription orders, though with triple the time when data had to be abstracted from medical records.

Problems encountered were frequent misspellings, the use of nonstandard abbreviations and, most seriously, prescriber lack of specificity. Assuming valid diagnosis information, criteria for diagnosis and drug match screening screened out 26.5 per cent of the prescription orders for intensive review, compared with 12.9 per cent for length of therapy and 12.0 per cent for dosage criteria. The dosage and therapy length screen had identified 787 prescription orders requiring attention; the addition of the diagnosis/drug screen detected an additional 703. Alternative screening criteria were established for the 10 drugs for which diagnosis was relevant to dosage or length of therapy, but only 4 per cent of the prescription orders for these drugs were for alternative diagnoses. An attempt to validate diagnosis information for antibiotics was unsuccessful because of inadequate laboratory data. Diagnosis validation remains the biggest unresolved problem. There is a danger that review, rather than improving drug usage, may induce prescriber recording of "appropriate" diagnoses. Accordingly, it seems best to begin a review system with criteria related to dosage and length of therapy, which are readily available and highly productive in identifying potential problems.

References, 4.

KNAPP, DAVID A.; BRANDON, BRENDA M.; KNAPP, DEANNE E.; KLEIN, LINDA S.; PALUMBO, FRANCIS B.; and SHAH, ROHIT. *Journal of the American Pharmaceutical Association NS 17* (2):103–106, February 1977.

Dollar Costs of Conducting Drug Use Review

134

The total direct costs for one drug use review in each of four settings, excluding the developmental costs of criteria and the computer program, ranged from $887 to $1,344, with the cost differential reflecting differences in the number of prescriptions sampled and the method of data collection.

Five categories of direct costs of conducting drug use review are identified and discussed: (1) development of screening criteria, (2) computer programming costs, (3) data collection costs, (4) data coding and processing costs, and (5) data analysis and reporting costs. Costs within each of the five categories are broken down into costs by specific function or service. Costs for the development of criteria for 50 drugs (40 adult and 10 pediatric) were $3,068. Computer programming costs totalled $3,333. Data collection costs depended on the data source used and varied from $117 to $644 per 1,000 prescription orders sampled. The specific data collection methods are discussed. Data coding and processing costs totalled $535.35 per thousand prescription orders.

Data analysis and report costs amounted to $290 per review. The indirect costs of drug use review are mentioned but not calculated.

References, 3.

KNAPP, DAVID A.; and PALUMBO, FRANCIS B. *Journal of the American Pharmaceutical Association NS17* (4):231–233, April 1977.

A Computer-Based Record and Clinical Monitoring System for Ambulatory Care

156 The Wishard Memorial Hospital in Indianapolis, Indiana, introduced in 1973 a computer-based record system as a supplement to a handwritten record system. This computer-based system automatically reminds physicians about significant clinical conditions of ambulatory care patients that may require action.

Physician orders (protocols) and patient medical records are stored in the computer, and protocols provide feedback to physicians to help improve medical care. For example, a typical protocol for detecting potential drug interactions reads: "If on Drug A and on Drug B, reduce dosage of A because . . ." Other types of protocol feedback remind physicians to adjust medication dosage if lab tests reveal certain conditions, to reconsider a particular medication because of a chronic condition, or to conduct a particular test if the last such test was performed too long ago or if certain conditions have been revealed by other tests. The computer project staff assists physicians in preparing these automatic standing orders.

Data worksheets include the Patient Encounter Form (medical history and orders), Patient Summary Report (showing clinical conditions over time), and Surveillance Report (presenting the actions suggested in the protocols). More than 200 health care personnel are using the system, which includes medical records for 7500 patients. Problems considered include data input mechanisms, paper records versus CRT displays, and the retrospective nature of the feedback.

An editorial appended to the article questions the long-term viability of a computer-assisted medical record system that relies partly on handwritten records.

References 2.

McDONALD, CLEMENT J.; MURRAY, RAYMOND; JERIS, DAVID; BHARGAVA, BHARAT; SEEGER, JAY; AND BLEVINS, LONNIE. *American Journal of Public Health 67* (3):240–245, March 1977.

Watching the Monitors: "PAID" Prescriptions, Fiscal Intermediaries and Drug Utilization Review

159 Because drug utilization review (DUR) and insurance claims review by financial administrative agencies such as PAID Prescriptions are undertaken for the purpose of saving money and only incidentally, if at all, for the purpose of improving physician prescribing habits, the PAID type of plan may not be the most appropriate mechanism for examining drug prescribing and dispensing practices.

The development of PAID Prescriptions is discussed, and the change from accepting "usual and customary" pharmacy fees to fixed fees is assessed. Incentives to change prescribing and dispensing practices may be found in capitation and risk acceptance plans, which stimulate interest in lower-cost drugs and increased efficiency. PAID's success in reducing costs for the San Joaquin Medi-Cal program has encouraged its use in several other states. However, it is suggested that these cost savings are easily explained because of the artificially high prices prevailing in the drug market; thus, any tightening of administrative controls on fees and processing costs was bound to save money.

PAID introduced a DUR committee of four pharmacists and one physician in the San Joaquin program in August 1970, to evaluate the prescriptions identified by the computerized system as failing to meet screening criteria, thus focusing attention on potential abuse of the system by patients, physicians and pharmacists.

References, 28.

MORGAN, JOHN P. *New England Journal of Medicine 296* (5):251–256, February 1977.

Detecting Prescribing Problems through Drug Usage Review: A Case Study

172

Retrospective review of more than 1000 prescription orders that included diagnostic data (for third-party payment) yielded information on prescribing problems such as mismatching diagnosis and prescribed drug, prescribing an inadequate dosage, insufficient or excessive length of drug therapy and inadequate labeling information for the patient. Criteria for length of therapy, dose and diagnosis were developed from the professional literature for 50 frequently prescribed drugs.

Prescription information was analyzed by computer. Of 1033 prescriptions, 56 per cent failed to pass one or more of the screens when compared with stated criteria. Mismatch between diagnosis and drug occurred in 23 per cent of the cases. Insufficient length of therapy occurred in 10 per cent of the cases, almost wholly with prescriptions for antibiotics. An automated retrospective drug utilization review system can identify potential prescribing problems, which may then be examined and acted upon by a drug use review committee.

References, 4.

PALUMBO, FRANCIS B.; KNAPP, DAVID A.; BRANDON, BRENDA M.; KNAPP, DEANNE E.; SOLOMON, DAVID K.; KLEIN, LINDA S.; and SHAH, ROHIT K. *American Journal of Hospital Pharmacy 34* (2):152–154, February 1977.

Conceptual Framework for Drug Usage Review, Medical Audit and Other Patient Care Review Procedures

233 The differences and interrelationships among seven topics are discussed: (1) quality assurance programs, (2) drug use review, (3) utilization review, (4) peer review, (5) medical audit, (6) patient care audit, and (7) medical care evaluation studies. A conceptual framework within which all hospital quality assurance mechanisms can be constructed is outlined. The theory and workings of a drug use review program are explained. The general role and specific duties of the hospital pharmacist in drug use review programs and peer review activities are discussed. Both programs are part of the pharmacy audit, which is one part of the overall patient care audit. Pharmaceutical services included in the peer review include drug distribution and control, drug information, clinical pharmacy and continuing education. Quality assurance programs and the pharmacist's role in one in a skilled nursing facility are briefly discussed.

References, 17. *Key words:* Inpatient settings.

STOLAR, MICHAEL H. *American Journal of Hospital Pharmacy* 34 (2):139–145, February 1977.

Drug Utilization Review in a Health Maintenance Organization. I. Introduction and Examples of Methodology

256 The institution of a drug utilization review program in the Columbia (Maryland) Medical Plan (a Health Maintenance Organization) brought about a decrease in prescriptions for antihistamines. Prescription drugs are covered by the prepaid plan if dispensed by the Plan pharmacy or authorized by the pharmacist to be dispensed elsewhere. Copayments are $2.00 for each prescription or refill. The Plan's Pharmacy and Therapeutics Committee developed criteria for seven major therapeutic categories, on the basis of an extensive literature review, for drug prescribing and dispensing practices; for example, restrictions on prescription size and appropriateness of a drug for a particular diagnosis. Drug use was reviewed before and after the criteria were approved.

Antihistamine data were chosen to illustrate the effects of the drug review. Criteria indicated that antihistamines should not be used for upper respiratory infections, and that single agent products should be used instead of more expensive combination products. Antihistamine prescriptions declined after adoption of the criteria from an average of 9.33 per 100 visits to 6.54 per 100 visits. The use of combination products did not change. One combination product was dropped from the formulary, but physicians prescribed another combination product instead.

The mechanisms for establishing prescribing criteria and for drug use review were shown to be satisfactory. The question is raised whether peer review should be used to discourage prescribing of a particular drug, or if the drug should simply be made unavailable by not including it in a formulary.

References, 13. *Key words:* Direct provision, formularies.

WEST, SHEILA K.; BRANDON, BRENDA M.; STEVENS, ANNE M.; ZAUBER, ANN; CHASE, GARY; STOLLEY, PAUL D.; and RUMRILL, RICHARD E. *Medical Care 15* (6):505–514, June 1977.

Drug Use Analysis Bibliography

259

This computer-generated 386-item bibliography on topics related to prescriber drug use provides citations to English language books, articles and research reports, as well as appropriate key words for each document. Author and subject lists are included. The bibliography was compiled by the Drug Use Analysis Branch of the FDA.

References, 386.

ZAX, BRIAN B.; and KNAPP, DEANNE E. Accession No. PB 264222/AS. Springfield, Virginia 22161, National Technical Information Service, March 1977.

1976

Constructing a Conceptual Model of Drug Utilization Review

31

A proposed framework for drug utilization review (DUR) programs, based on 5 principles, is easily applicable to institutional settings such as hospitals, clinics and Health Maintenance Organizations. These principles are: (1) to be legitimate, utilization review must be based on recognized authority; (2) the interpretation of drug use patterns must consider the distinguishing characteristics of the health services providers and the patient population (for example, physicians' specialties, hospital affiliations and ages, patients' ages, income levels and levels of education, all influence drug prescribing and use patterns); (3) utilization and cost data must be available to establish a baseline drug profile with which developments can be compared over time; (4) appropriate criteria and standards for prescribing, dispensing and using drugs must be established; (5) short-term (perhaps annual) drug use studies to investigate possible changes in factors such as consumption, costs, adverse drug reactions, utilization of selected classes of drugs, under and over utilization, and third party expenditures, must be part of a comprehensive DUR program.

The model is less immediately applicable to noninstitutional ambulatory care, because of the lack of a defined population of patients and providers, the lack of a central data organization and systematic or standardized record-keeping by physicians and pharmacists, and the tendency to obtain prescriptions from more than one physician concurrently. Other issues in DUR are costs (especially where automated equipment is involved) and the delicate relationship between physician and pharmacist.

References, 17. *Key words:* Inpatient settings.

BRODIE, DONALD C.; and SMITH, WILLIAM E. *Hospitals 50* (6):143–144, 146, 148, 150, March 1976.

Effect of Medical Care Review on the Use of Injections

33

In 1971 the Health and Social Services Department of New Mexico, the New Mexico Foundation for Medical Care and the Dikewood Corporation, joined to develop a system for claims processing and for reviewing the quality of services rendered within the New Mexico Medicaid program. This study focused primarily on the quality of use of injections given to the New Mexico Medicaid population between September 1, 1971 and August 31, 1973.

It was found that current review could affect certain quality aspects of the program, in particular the appropriateness of the use of injections as judged by medical criteria. Nearly 50 per cent of the injections in this study were antibiotics, and their use declined by more than 60 per cent, from 41 to 16 per 100 ambulatory visits. However, at the end of the study, 40 per cent of the injections administered were considered medically unnecessary.

Analysis of the data led to two major findings: (1) groups of physicians used injections more appropriately than solo physicians and (2) for solo physicians, being board certified, being a pediatrician or being a doctor of medicine were associated with the more proper use of injections. Additionally, it was found that 22 physicians (6 per cent) gave 41 per cent of the inappropriate injections in the program and provided only 13.5 per cent of the ambulatory visits. As a result of the current review system, these physicians changed their behavior substantially for the better.

References, 17.

BROOK, ROBERT H.; and WILLIAMS, KATHLEEN N. A study of the New Mexico experimental medical care review organization. *Annals of Internal Medicine* 85 (4):509–515, October 1976.

State-of-the-Art of Drug Usage Review

89

Analysis of 22 drug use review (DUR) studies from medical, allied health and pharmaceutical journals (1970–1975) revealed deficiencies in content and methodology, such as implicit rather than explicit standards and lack of sampling and screening criteria, which lead to slow and subjective or unreliable reviews. More objective standards and procedures permit DUR to be undertaken by community pharmacies or small health facilities by technical staff, conserving the time of professional personnel for indepth review. Additional problems noted were that (1) most DUR was retrospective (this is simpler than concurrent or prospective DUR, but is not of immediate benefit to patients); (2) antibiotics were the most frequently studied drug class, to the exclusion of other classes; (3) feedback should be provided to the physician if DUR is to result in improved prescribing practices. DUR of prescribing practices was defined as including systematic data collection of prescription orders and evaluation of these orders on daily dose, length of therapy or quantity dispensed, or appropriateness of the drug itself. Data are also reported on components of DUR relating to standards and review procedures (personnel, facilities, computer usage, sampling, follow-up, financing).

References, 6.

GREGORY, JOHN M.; and KNAPP, DEANNE E. *American Journal of Hospital Pharmacy* 33 (9):925–928, September 1976.

Physicians' Responses to Peer Review and Drug Utilization Review Procedures of a Medicaid Drug Program

147

The drug utilization review (DUR) mechanism of the Florida Medicaid drug program, administered by PAID Prescriptions, was assessed after one year of operation and was shown to have significantly reduced drug expenditures in 39 per cent of the cases examined. Eight regional committees, each consisting of four pharmacists and two physicians, reviewed patient drug profiles that exceeded one or more of the following monthly criteria: $50.00, eight claims, prescriptions from three physicians, or four purchases within one therapeutic class. Letters were sent to physicians requesting diagnoses, evaluation and recommendations for improving the patient's drug therapy, and an indication of whether the physician was aware of the patient's exceptional drug use.

Of the 4700 physicians contacted throughout 1975, 68 per cent responded to the DUR committee letters. Fifteen per cent of the replies indicated an intention of changing the patient's medication. A six-month follow-up was made of these patients and the average saving per patient was found to be $99.00. Potential savings through this review program are estimated at 2 per cent of annual benefits. The DUR committees plan to improve profile review and physician follow-up procedures and to familiarize greater numbers of physicians with the purpose of DUR. This should lead to greater savings.

References, 0.

LEROY, A.A.; MORSE, M.L.; and McCORMICK, W.C. Jacksonville, Florida, PAID Prescriptions, 1976.

Drug Use Analysis Methodologies

135

A system designed to alert the Food and Drug Administration to instances of overprescribing of certain drugs was tested with Medicaid outpatients in California (72 patients receiving the drug meperidine) and North Carolina (455 patients receiving phenmetrazine) during 1975. Prescriptions were examined for daily dose, days supply, length of therapy and total number of prescriptions per patient. Criteria were developed against which to compare current prescribing practices in order to determine the incidence of overprescribing. The criteria, developed from the professional literature and professional expertise, were considered liberal. The methodology for data collection and analysis is presented.

For meperidine, only 1 per cent of the 176 prescriptions exceeded the criteria on days supply and daily dose. For phenmetrazine, 3 per cent of the 820 prescriptions exceeded these criteria. The screening methodology is considered cost effective. It is not necessary that each prescription be examined; rather, large numbers of prescriptions can be reviewed rapidly to see where prescribing problems may lie. Another methodology was applied to national data for nonrefillable drugs from the *National Prescription Audit* in an attempt to forecast prescribing patterns.

References, 7.

KNAPP, DEANNE E.; CROSBY, DIANNE L.; MORGAN, THOMAS F.; LAO, CHANG S.; KENNEDY, J. STEPHEN; and DORMER, ROBERT A. Accession No. PB 260542/AS. Springfield, Virginia 22161, National Technical Information Service, 1976.

Drug Utilization Review. Current Status and Relationship to Assuring Quality Medical Care

136

In 1974, total expenditures for prescription drugs were approximately 11 billion dollars, or greater than 10 per cent of the total cost of medical care services. The magnitude of drug use in medical practice today is obviously considerable. Because of the large utilization of prescription drugs, there is a great deal of concern on the part of third-party payers to contain drug cost. There is evidence that the prescribing habits of physicians are poor and are probably contributing to high drug use. In addition, drug utilization is expected to increase in the years ahead, thereby requiring cost and quality control mechanisms, such as drug utilization review (DUR) or peer review.

This paper presents an overview of the current status of DUR and its relationship to the assurance of quality medical care. Most United States systems are retrospective in nature and are based on screening drug claims by comparing drug prescribing to criteria of drug use. These criteria are commonly based on quantity standards of appropriateness. The primary deficiency of current DUR programs is the relative lack of measures of quality. Secondly, there exists a need to integrate drug use review into the overall medical care review process. This paper presents recommendations for demonstration and research efforts.

References, 48.

KNOBEN, JAMES E. *Drug Intelligence and Clinical Pharmacy 10* (4):222–228, April 1976.

Antibiotic Use Control—An Institutional Model

180

This paper describes: (1) the development and implementation of an institutional program of antibiotic use control cosponsored by a Pharmacy and Therapeutics Committee and an Infection Control Committee; (2) the application and genesis of a practical methodology for both prospective and retrospective institutional antibiotic drug use review (DUR); and (3) the results of a retrospective review of cephalosporin use in 102 hospitalized patients over a 12-month period.

The antibiotic DUR program includes a formal educational program and in-house controls on the use of certain antibiotics. The two committees have established rigid controls on the use of expensive, highly selective, or potentially toxic antibiotics. Regarding this latter category, house staff physicians prescribing them must have such orders countersigned by a representative of the Infection Control Committee.

Of the 102 patients for whom antibiotic use was studied, 49 per cent were designated as having received cephalosporin derivatives rationally for the treatment of active infectious disease or prophylaxis. The remaining patients received therapy that was judged to be irrational or questionable, according to the criteria set up for the study. Also discussed in this paper is prospective

DUR, using clinical pharmacy services and clinical microbiology monitoring systems.

References, 40. *Key words:* Inpatient settings.

PIERPAOLI, PAUL G.; COARSE, JAMES F.; and TILTON, RICHARD C. *Drug Intelligence and Clinical Pharmacy 10* (5):258–267, May 1976.

An Eclectic Approach to Quality Control in Fee-for-Service Health Care: The New York City Medicaid Experience

188

A computer system (Medicaid Vendor System or MVS) designed to evaluate individual provider deficiencies in the New York City Medicaid program is described. The system has been used to profile all services rendered since 1973. The MVS system is an interim program for use during the development of a more sophisticated system. Three reports are produced by MVS: (1) individual profiles for each fee-for-service provider, (2) statistical profiles for each provider type, thus permitting norms of services of Medicaid providers to be established, and (3) exception reports or listings of providers whose billed services exceed predetermined limits relating to the distribution of service codes on their individual profiles (e.g., a time constraint parameter would be the number of patient visits per day).

The providers flagged in the exception reports are investigated further for possible abuses of the Medicaid system. Exception report summaries are compiled in order to set priorities for further investigation. Many methods are used to investigate suspected abuses; e.g., personal interviews of patients and/or providers, collection of physical evidence such as pill containers.

The evaluation program led to three conclusions: (1) many providers were guilty of fiscal abuse or of providing deficient health care, (2) no single evaluation technique can answer all questions, and (3) the deviation-from-norm approach is a very useful method of evaluation. Implications of the evaluation program for Professional Standards Review Organizations and national health insurance are discussed.

References, 23.

ROSENBERG, STEPHEN N., GUNSTON, CHRISTINE; BERENSON, LOUISE; and KLEIN, ARLETTE. *American Journal of Public Health 66* (*1*):21–30, January 1976.

Computer Support of Pharmaceutical Services for Ambulatory Patients

253

The computer-based support system for the ambulatory pharmacy services of the Appalachian Regional Hospitals is described. Appalachian Regional Hospitals is a rural health care system consisting of ten hospitals and several primary care centers. The outpatient pharmacies dispense 1300 prescriptions per day. All patients are members of a third-party program which pays only for drugs for chronic diseases. Diagnosis is required on the prescription and a formulary is used.

A technical description of the electronic data processing system is provided. A Univac 9480 central processing unit is used, plus miscellaneous other hardware. Eleven display units and three printers are available in the pharmacies. The system contains 20 data files and can recall patient records on-line.

In operation, a nonpharmacist enters prescription information into the system. A prescription label is typed automatically and the drugs selected and packaged. At this point, a pharmacist checks the patient records for any potential problems before dispensing. The system is capable of carrying out retrospective review. This has been accomplished only to a limited extent to date. Several general tables are provided on the number of prescriptions per patient, the number of diagnoses per prescription, the number of prescriptions by physician and the top twenty drugs and therapeutic categories. No explicit criteria are used in the retrospective review and, to date, no prescribing profiles for individual physicians have been generated.

A summary of the results of prospective review of over 115,000 new prescriptions is presented. Approximately 2.2 per cent of the total prescriptions had a potential problem which was detected by the computer system.

References, 9. *Key words:* Formularies

WEISSMAN, ALAN M.; SOLOMON, DAVID K.; BAUMGARTNER, R. PAUL, JR.; BRADY, JEFFREY A.; PETERSON, JAMES H.; and KNIGHT, JOSEPH L. *American Journal of Hospital Pharmacy 33 (11)*:1171–1175, November 1976.

1975

Professional Standards Review Organizations—Participation Pathways for Pharmacists

100

Assuming that the still untried Professional Standards Review Organizations (PSROs) are necessary and can be made to succeed if their built-in defects—lack of interdisciplinary review in an era of interdisciplinary team delivery of health care and the conflict of interest in a physician only structure—are eliminated, there are ways pharmacists should help make them work. Increasing rational drug use is prerequisite to more adequate health care. It cannot be achieved through physician education because of vested interests, drug company competitiveness and an irreversible trend toward specialization. It makes sense to turn to the clinical pharmacist for a solution, and the PSRO offers a medium for bringing his expertise into the mainstream of medical review.

Pharmacists can participate via three interdependent approaches: joining advisory groups that will serve state PSRO Councils, getting one's hospital designated a "delegated review" facility and developing pharmacist-oriented concurrent review there, and working for PSRO structural changes. The latter will be politically difficult but is of crucial importance to the future of clinical pharmacy practice, because control of review means control of practices. While the first two approaches are short-term holding actions, they should be pursued aggressively to ensure that PSRO guidelines permitting participation by providers of ancillary services are liberally interpreted. Successful interdisciplinary review hinges on tactfully winning physicians over to viewing patient health status as a common reference point. Quickest results can probably be obtained by pharmacists working to get delegated review status for truly qualified hospitals. The pharmacy and therapeutic committee presents a good vehicle for drug utilization review and communication about appropriate drug usage. The trend toward stronger authority for these existing committees should be strengthened. Even greater impact can be had through the more immediate role of the clinical pharmacy service. It should be working routinely with the prescriber—supported by strong information systems and as something more than a drug distribution system—to promote rational drug therapy.

References, 4.

HIRSCHMAN, JOSEPH L.; and LAVENTURIER, MARC. *Drug Intelligence and Clinical Pharmacy 9* (*10*):553–556, October 1975.

Drug Utilization Review of Medicaid Patients: Therapeutic Implications and Opportunities

105

A North Carolina drug utilization review program under Medicaid examines, monthly, computer printouts of recipient drug purchases for prescription duplication, overutilization and drug interactions, and has brought about a reduction in drug costs. It was found unfeasible to screen for noncompliance. Most studies dealing with adverse drug reactions have involved hospital patients; little attention has been paid to the problem with nonhospitalized patients. Treating adverse drug reactions costs approximately $3 billion a year. Of such reactions, 70–80 per cent can be avoided by utilizing information on patient history and drug action. Therefore, care in drug selection and surveillance of drug use are indicated. PAID Prescriptions, administering the North Carolina Title XIX Medicaid program for prescription drug benefits, runs a drug utilization review program in which six pharmacists and one physician in each of four regions meet monthly. They inform local physicians and pharmacists by letter of unnecessary or inefficient drug use (including the patient's drug profile and information on possible drug interaction). Feedback will be requested, but the program's primary goal is to provide the information.

References, 13.

HULL, J. HEYWARD; BROWN, H. SHELTON; YARBOROUGH, FRANK F. and MURRAY, WILLIAM J. *North Carolina Medical Journal 36* (*3*):162–163, March 1975.

Incorporating Diagnosis into Drug Use Review Systems

129

This study was supported by the American Pharmaceutical Association through the Office of Economic Opportunity (OEO) project on the delivery of pharmaceutical services for ambulatory care programs. It emphasized drug use review activities which incorporate diagnosis or intended drug use information into the data base. Prescribing data were collected and analyzed at four sites (1974–1975) and reports made to pharmacists for use in drug utilization review programs. Sites included: (1) a neighborhood health center, located in the downtown area of a large northeastern city and handling approximately 2500 new prescriptions per month (diagnosis information was included on all prescriptions); (2) an outpatient pharmacy in a rural hospital in a mid-Atlantic state, handling approximately 450 new and renewal prescriptions per day (75 per cent of the prescriptions were paid for by third-party programs requiring diagnosis or intended drug use information on prescriptions); (3) a small ambulatory care clinic in rural Appalachia, handling approximately 35 prescriptions per day from orders on patient charts; (4) an Indian Health Service pharmacy, handling approximately 45,000 new prescriptions per year from orders in medical records.

Criteria were established for: acceptable indications for use, maximum and minimum daily dosage, maximum and minimum quantities (representing length of therapy). Underdosing was found more frequently than overdosing, especially with antibiotics. Ways of organizing drug use data for review are considered, along with major direct costs of the review system. The study concluded that a drug use review system working from diagnosis information on prescription orders is feasible, and can be accomplished manually. A quarterly retrospective review cycle is recommended. Appendices contain data collection instructions, drug use screening criteria for adults and children, results of drug use review, site visits and presentations by staff.

References, four page bibliography.

KNAPP, DAVID A.; BRANDON, BRENDA M.; KNAPP, DEANNE E.; KLEIN, LINDA S.; and PALUMBO, FRANCIS B. Final Report. Office of Economic Opportunity Project No. 31617. Baltimore, University of Maryland School of Pharmacy, 1975.

The Professional Standards Review Organization Program—Its Impact on the Provision of Drug-Related Services

137

There are two aspects of the Professional Standards Review Organization (PSRO) program with which the pharmacist can be involved: (1) in an advisory capacity and in the review of the quality of health care services and (2) in the determination of the medical necessity and appropriateness (i.e., utilization) of health care services. PSRO legislation requires that each Statewide Professional Standards Review Council or each PSRO in states without statewide councils shall be assisted by an Advisory Group, which shall consist of physician and nonphysician health care practitioners (e.g., pharmacist). Through the pharmacist's participation in the Advisory Group, PSROs and statewide councils can be kept apprised of current developments within the pharmacy field.

The role of the pharmacist in PSRO review involves peer review of pharmacy practice and chemotherapy review. The development of model standards and criteria for professional practice relating to each of these two aspects is required on a national level. The pharmacist can be involved in the development of criteria and standards for and in the actual review of drug-related medical care evaluation studies. Finally, the pharmacist can be involved in continuing education programs for health professionals on proper drug therapy. In the drug utilization aspect of PSRO review, the pharmacist can have an important role in the development of model PSRO drug utilization review programs. Four model systems, currently under joint development by the IMS America Corporation and the Commission on Professional and Hospital Activities, are scheduled for completion in late 1976.

References, 3.

KNOBEN, JAMES E. *Journal of the American Pharmaceutical Association NS15 (11)*:614–615, 644, November 1975.

Drug Use Data: A Different Perspective

142

Even though T. Donald Rucker is correct in stressing drug utilization review as a means to improved therapy, his article in the *Journal of the American Medical Association 230*:888–890, 1974 calling for a national computerized drug data bank with terminals in every pharmacy is a clear case of overkill. Since drugs actually account for a steadily declining share of health care expenditures, potential cost savings from utilization review cannot compare with economies from avoiding unnecessary hospitalization. Dr. Rucker claims a $600 million information system would be cost-beneficial because preventable adverse drug reactions (ADRs) cost an estimated $4 billion a year. He arrived at this preposterously high estimate in an earlier article by adding costs of an estimated 30,000 ADR-induced deaths to estimates of $3 billion to $3.6 billion for hospital care for ADR reactions, some 70–80 per cent of which are "predictable, hence preventable."

Following through on footnotes and citations eventually leads to a misreading or improper extrapolation of data from the Boston Collaborative Drug Surveillance Study as the main source of death and hospitalization estimates. One writer pointed out ways the numbers were manipulated, e.g., by blaming drugs for cancer patient deaths, and the Boston group's spokesman has interpreted the data as suggesting unnecessary drug toxicity only in the area of fluid and electrolyte therapy. It is hard to see how a computer network could prevent ADRs from intravenous administration or cancer chemotherapy. Every physician obviously has to make an individual cost-benefit judgement to treat a seriously ill patient.

Dr. Rucker's exaggeration of the extent of both drug use ($8 billion seems a more accurate estimate for 1973 than his $11 billion) and the incidence and cost of ADRs implies a crisis situation calling for drastic government intervention. His proposal at a time of general budgetary stringency to invest $600 million in a computer network connecting all physicians and pharmacists to a government bureaucracy certainly requires rigorous cost-benefit analysis.

References, 7.

See abstract 192, p. 190.

LEE, ARMISTEAD M. *Journal of the American Medical Association 234 (12)*:1242–1244, December 22, 1975.

Drug Utilization in the Hospital: An Evaluation of Drug Costs

153

Cost data for 9 common drug groups administered to 7423 general medical service inpatients (August 1, 1969—March 13, 1973) show that certain drug groups were responsible for a disproportionate share of hospital pharmacy costs. The average number of drugs administered to each patient was 8.04. The average annual cost of drugs for the 9 index drug groups administered during the study period was $24,948, half the total drug costs for these patients. Demographic data on patients were obtained from hospital admission forms. Data on drugs administered were recorded on special medication forms and processed by computer. Cost data were obtained from the hospital pharmacy and from state contracts.

The 3 most expensive index drug groups (6 antimicrobial, 4 anti-inflammatory, 2 anticoagulant) accounted for 81 per cent of the total cost of all drug groups studied, but only 22 per cent of the total patient exposures to the drugs studied. The 3 least expensive drug groups (5 analgesic, 4 antiarrhythmic, 4 sedative-tranquilizer) accounted for 11 per cent of the cost (and the lowest average per patient cost) and 62 per cent of the patient exposures. The other drug groups (3 antihypertensive, 3 diuretic, 3 antacid) accounted for 8 per cent of the cost and 16 per cent of the patient exposures. Cost, utilization and dosage data are presented for each drug in these groups. Reducing costs of the 3 most expensive drug groups studied by 10 per cent would result in an 8 per cent cost reduction over all drug groups.

Utilization of some drugs declined during the study period when new drugs were introduced (some at higher costs and some at lower costs). Changes in dosage form also affected costs, as did drugs which required laboratory tests and frequent patient monitoring. Drug utilization review is recommended to assess both patient welfare and hospital expenditures.

References, 16.

MAY, FRANKLIN E.; STEWART, RONALD B.; and CLUFF, LEIGHTON E. *Drugs in Health Care* 2 (3):139–152, Summer 1975.

Professional Standards Review Organizations: An Opportunity for Pharmacy

219 The establishment of Professional Standards Review Organizations (PSROs) became law in October 1972. PSROs are local nonprofit groups of physicians who evaluate the necessity and quality of medical care in their geographic area, based on accepted standards of practice. Initially affecting federal Medicare and Medicaid programs, PSROs are included in all pending national health insurance legislation. HEW steps to implement the law in 203 PSRO areas are described, including guidelines and instructions from the *PSRO Manual.* Applications from physician organizations seeking participation in the PSRO program are of 3 types: (1) planning contracts, (2) conditional contracts (assistance for organizations ready to implement PSROs), and (3) statewide support center contracts (assistance for newly formed PSROs in administrative, organizational and professional matters). PSRO activities include review of drug utilization and pharmaceutical services as part of quality control in the provision of drug products. A clear professional relationship between pharmacist and physician must be defined. Pharmacists are eligible to serve on PSRO advisory boards, but physicians are responsible for final decision making.

Drug utilization review programs are usually retrospective, dealing with drug type, dose, quantity and frequency of prescription in various therapeutic categories. Additional criteria should be included in PSRO programs: the patient's medical problem or medical purpose for which the drug is ordered, other drugs the patient is taking which may interact with the prescribed drug or be inappropriate, and laboratory tests with which the prescribed drug may interfere. Pharmacists should be involved in developing standards for professional practice through national interdisciplinary efforts, developing guidelines for the conduct of peer review and of medical education relating to drug utilization, and assisting the local or state PSRO.

References, 0.

SIMMONS, HENRY E. *Drugs in Health Care* 2 (*1*):3–7, Winter 1975.

1974

Pharmacist-Monitored, Computerized Drug Usage Review

109

The computerized pharmacy drug usage review program at the Montefiore Hospital and Medical Center is discussed. Five drugs in thirteen dosage forms are currently under review; the program could be expanded to include all formulary drugs. The five steps of pharmacy data input and the functional operations of the computer program are discussed in detail. A weekly report of patient drug usage profiles and a monthly report of drug usage by hospital service are currently produced. Special reports can be compiled as needed. During its year of operation, the program has generated sufficient information for the development of drug usage guidelines. The impact of the program on drug usage and control will be assessed in the future.

References, 9. *Key words:* Inpatient settings.

JACINTO, MARCIA S.; KLEINMANN, KURT; and MARGOLIN, JOSEPH, *American Journal of Hospital Pharmacy* 31 (5):508–512, May 1974.

Development and Application of Criteria in Drug Use Review Programs

132

The essential components of the drug use process are identified in order to develop objective criteria for drug utilization review. A specific set of criteria, developed by the staff of the University of Maryland School of Pharmacy for reviewing certain aspects of drug use for sixty-five common drugs, is set forth. A sample set of criteria for one set of data related to antibiotic therapy is discussed. The definitions of terms and concepts associated with drug use review and used by the Office of Professional Standards Review are presented in detail. Six steps of the drug use and prescription process are discussed in relation to the norms, criteria and standards which have previously been applied at each step.

The six stages are: (1) determining the need for a drug, (2) selection of specific drug products, (3) selection of regimen, (4) obtaining the drug product, (5) administration/consumption of the drug products and (6) effect of drug therapy. The authors stress that the establishment of health care quality assurance programs depends upon the systematic development of objective criteria of drug use.

References, 15, plus 22 in appendix.

KNAPP, DAVID A.; KNAPP, DEANNE E.; BRANDON, BRENDA M.; and WEST, SHEILA. *American Journal of Hospital Pharmacy 31* (7):648–656, July 1974.

Drug Use. Data, Sources and Limitations

192 A national drug information system clearing house is described as a means of ensuring the privacy of patient-care considerations over economic considerations in the implementation of national health insurance. The system would record and retrieve data for clinical, administrative, educational and research needs relating to drug use, and be compatible with a future general health care information network.

Pharmacists would record prescriptions dispensed on terminals and the information would be transmitted to regional computer centers for analysis and storage (the clearing houses). In the future, terminals could be placed in physicians' offices for more direct transmission of prescription orders (to be retrieved and dispensed by pharmacists). Clearing houses would develop drug and patient profiles and would transmit third-party insurance claims. Professional access to data would be free of time constraints. In one proposed system, clinicians could conduct a concurrent review of prescription options and problems while the patient was being treated.

Costs of a national drug information network are estimated at "well under" $600 million annually; expected annual savings exceed $4 billion. One risk is the likelihood that third-party interests, and not patient and professional needs, would govern system and operation. Sources of data for the information system include the United States Bureau of Census and the Pharmaceutical Manufacturers Association (production data), the National Center for Health Statistics and the Social Security Administration (data on drug use) and studies conducted by organizations such as the National Institutes of Mental Health. However, much information is out of date or unavailable. The acquisition of comprehensive and current prescription information is vital to support patient care, therefore a national information system should be considered.

References, 24.

See abstract 142, p. 187.

RUCKER, T. DONALD. *Journal of the American Medical Association 230* (6):888–890, November 11, 1974.

1973

Medicaid Drug Program Utilization Study

108 This study of the functioning of the Iowa Medicaid Drug Program found that, with peer review and utilization control, a favorable cost-benefit ratio can be maintained in a relatively unrestricted pharmaceutical benefits program. Included is an analysis and evaluation of computerized data from the Medicaid program covering pharmaceutical services for October 1, 1970 to March 13,

1971. The recommendations are for: continuing peer review and utilization control activities; continued attention to recipients identified as heavy users of pharmaceuticals (which could result from incomplete records and thus poor supervision of drug therapy); prescribing a full month's supply of medication for chronic illness (fewer prescriptions reduce the number of Medicaid fees); recording physician instructions on drug use in a data bank to facilitate utilization review; coding all drug products for computer use; and recording the patient's diagnosis on the claims form.

The study includes statistical data on 102,517 persons eligible for Medicaid and provides reports on health care costs by type of health service provider and major aid category, as well as average prescription cost and quantity dispensed. It discusses ways to make meaningful state-by-state comparison of Medicaid statistics. Profiles of 5751 patient records for persons who received drugs which cost more than $120.00 during the six-month study are provided, and problems such as "doctor shopping," long periods of medication without re-examination and multiple drug products supplied to patients on a recurring basis are reported. Psychotropic drugs account for 17.67 per cent of total dollar expenditures for drug purchases; this cost is considered preferable, economically, to paying for alternative hospitalization and treatment.

References, 14.

IOWA DEPARTMENT OF SOCIAL SERVICES. Des Moines, Bureau of Medical Services, 1973.

The Restrictive Formulary and Drug Use Review in a Medicare Out-of-Hospital Prescription Drug Program

127

The restrictive formulary and drug use review are discussed in relation to three requirements of an out-of-hospital Medicare drug program: (1) assurance of drug product quality, (2) assurance of the quality of drug use, and (3) cost control. In a restrictive federal formulary, only the "best available" drug products would presumably be listed, thereby insuring drug quality and lowered drug costs. The role of the Food and Drug Administration (FDA) in assuring drug quality is discussed. In comparison with a restrictive formulary, the FDA is viewed as the better vehicle to assure drug quality for all Americans. Reasons why drug use review is viewed as a better method than the restrictive formulary for preventing inappropriate (over-, under-, or mis-prescribing) drug use are discussed. The need to establish criteria for optimal drug use and the level of acceptable variation in advance of review in order to evaluate empirical data is discussed. Drug use review would need to be established and implemented on a local level, with federal and state guidance. The Professional Standards Review Organization system should include a requirement for drug use review. Neither drug use review nor a restrictive formulary are viewed as the appropriate means to control the costs of drug therapy.

References, 11.

KNAPP, DAVID A. *National Association of Retail Druggists Journal 95* (20):14–16, October 15, 1973.

Drug Use Review—A Manual System

131 A simple and inexpensive system of drug use review, which has been tested in 5 diverse Office of Economic Opportunity Neighborhood Health Centers, is outlined. It enables small health programs to begin getting a picture of prescribing patterns, as a step toward efficiently optimizing the quality of drug therapy. Features of the system are that it requires no extra personnel or electronic data processing equipment, can be used in an in-house or vendor program, derives data by sampling dispensed prescription orders, offers model criteria for 50 common drugs, and provides for local review and analysis.

A technician samples 15–20 prescription orders a day, copies the drug name and strength, quantity dispensed, directions, renewal instructions, name of the prescriber and prescription number onto specially prepared data cards, and codes the name of the prescriber and guideline drugs by notching the edge of the card with a hand punch. Every few weeks, the pharmacist in charge runs a sorting needle through the edge-notched cards to group them by drug code. He then compares the cards with guidelines for minimum and maximum doses and quantities, which reflect expert opinion and which the professional staff supports.

Since a prescription may fall outside criteria limits for valid reasons, the pharmacist sometimes consults a patient's medical record. He uses his judgment for uncoded drugs. A second sort places the cards in groups by prescriber code and by drug within groups. The pharmacist next prepares a summary table showing, by prescriber in rows and by drugs in columns, the numbers of total prescriptions, and of prescriptions outside the criteria. He writes a report analyzing the table from the standpoints of patterns of use by the center, by individual prescriber and by drugs with many prescriptions outside criteria. The report is presented to a drug use review committee composed of center professional personnel. This committee, perhaps after calling on the pharmacist for further information, determines if any remedial action, such as education or policy-setting, is warranted.

References, 6.

KNAPP, DAVID A.; BRANDON, BRENDA M.; WEST, SHEILA; and LEAVITT, DEAN E. *Journal of the American Pharmaceutical Association NS13* (8):417–420, 433, August 1973.

Drug Utilization Review by Pharmacy and Therapeutics Committees

182 The major goal of the national Drug Spotlight Program is to help hospital pharmacy and therapeutics committees improve rational drug therapy. This program is conducted by several hospital, medical, pharmacy and nursing groups.

The program will "spotlight" four groups of drugs, the first of which are antihypertension agents. Three possible areas of participation by the hospital pharmacist are: (1) periodic review of established physicial and laboratory parameters to assess the course of the disease and monitoring of the patient's progress through therapy, (2) development and promotion of programs to fight hypertension, and (3) screening of patients for hypertension.

References, 0. *Key words:* Inpatient settings.

REILLY, MARY JO. *American Journal of Hospital Pharmacy 30* (4):349–350, April 1973.

Professional Standards Review Organizations and Pharmacy

197

The 1972 legislation requiring that Professional Standards Review Organizations (PSROs), representing areas to be designated and composed of a majority of the area's physicians, be set up nationwide to evaluate Medicare and Medicaid claims is of extreme significance to health care and to pharmacy. The goals are to ensure that services are medically necessary and meet professionally recognized standards and to identify cheaper ways of providing some institutional care. State and local review councils will have coordinating roles and a National Professional Standards Review Council will guide, provide technical assistance and evaluate. Appropriate professionals will assist in the local development of norms of care.

The PSROs will maintain profiles on providers and patients and report divergences between standards and patterns of care. Measures are included to protect confidentiality, provide against conflicts of interest, allow appeals and assuage fears about malpractice claims. The enabling legislation never mentions drugs or pharmacy. However, PSROs have jurisdiction over "services for which payment may be made under the Social Security Act" and this amounted to $1.49 billion in prescription services in 1971. It also seems likely that regulations will eventually include pharmacy services, because prescribing practices are part of a physician's profile. Patient profiles cover all "care and services" and providers other than physicians are to be reviewed. Pharmacists cannot participate in final review determination, but may help establish standards for rational prescribing, participate in initial interview and perhaps serve on advisory committees to the state review councils.

Professional organizations have seldom led in demanding quality assurance procedures. In the past, insurance programs have asked their help only with problems of overutilization, and criteria have tended to be too gross to distinguish appropriate from inappropriate care (e.g., across-the-board day limits for drug quantities). The new system also faces difficult administrative problems, like keeping massive data up-to-date, holding costs down, and operating across different jurisdictional lines from multiple carriers. Considering the volume of prescription claims to be evaluated and the importance of physician productivity, a system for concurrent review seems vital and a computerized system separating evaluation and compensation ought to be devised.

Pharmacist associations and the American Association of Colleges of Pharmacy are going to have to select review participants and devise specialized training programs for participants, who must focus on jointly optimizing patient care, rather than get into conflicts with physicians over who should evaluate drug therapy. The dilemma that norm-setting by peers can perpetuate poor practices, while deference to experts can jeopardize general cooperation, will hopefully be minimized by the provisions for regional standard setting, ranges of acceptable care and national guidance. Modifying problem practitioner behavior will probably work best if permitted educational efforts focus on the scientific basis for a standard.

References, 19.

RUCKER, T. DONALD. *Journal of the American Pharmaceutical Association NS13* (*10*):568–570, 591, October 1973.

Use of Laboratory Tests and Pharmaceuticals. Variation among Physicians and Effect of Cost Audit on Subsequent Use

207 This study of the patterns of physician utilization of laboratory tests and prescription behavior revealed that great variation existed among physicians in costs of laboratory and drug use, a 17-fold variation in laboratory costs and a 4-fold variation in drug costs. Physician knowledge of the results of the cost audit resulted in a 29.2 per cent decrease in laboratory costs ($p < .01$) and a 6.4 per cent increase in drug expenditures ($p < .01$).

The physicians studied were 33 faculty internists. Ten to fifteen patients per physician where chosen at random from among those patients meeting certain eligibility requirements, e.g., to have from 2 to 8 of the medical problems on a "Master Problem List." No effort was made to study comparable groups, in terms of demographic and clinical characteristics, of the patients. All laboratory and drug charges for each patient during a three-month period in 1971 were totaled and calculated on an annual basis. Mean annual laboratory and drug costs for each physician's patients were calculated.

Each physician was informed of his ranking (in terms of his patients' laboratory and drug expenditures) relative to other physicians. The study was repeated for a second three-month period in order to assess how physician behavior in ordering laboratory tests and prescribing drugs changed as a result of the cost audit. Several physician variables, e.g., physician age, internal medicine board certification, were analyzed; there was no significant correlation between any of the physician variables and costs of care. The relative cost behavior of the physicians was generally consistent during the six-month period. The study did not attempt to measure quality of health care, nor attempt to obtain information relating cost to either quality or efficiency of medical care.

References, 6.

SCHROEDER, STEVEN A.; KENDERS, KATHRYN; COOPER, JAMES K.; and PIEMME, THOMAS E. *Journal of the American Medical Association 225* (8):969–973, August 20, 1973.

1972

Drug Utilization Review with On-Line Computer Capability. Selected Methodology and Findings from a Demonstration

150 This project at Los Angeles County-University of Southern California (LAC-USC) Medical Center, described by Maronde, stands almost alone as an operating model of drug use review in an ambulatory setting. In the relatively controlled environment of LAC-USC, over five years and $2 million in grant and contract funds were expended to reach the point described in the book. At LAC-USC, pharmacists in the clinic assist the physician in drug choice decisions and have been delegated full authority to determine the quantities to be prescribed. Since a formulary is used at the Center, a therapeutics committee determines the choice of suppliers. Clerical personnel are used to input data into patient drug histories and to type prescription labels.

Maronde and his colleagues started with the prescribed drug therapy of the Medical Center's 700 physicians. Drug use was already controlled or limited to a certain extent by a formulary containing 1400 drugs. Only a fraction of one per cent of all drugs used at the Center are nonformulary items. The 700 physicians care for an outpatient population of about 200,000 individuals. The site of care is the outpatient clinic of the LAC-USC Medical Center. Pharmacies in the clinic and in the main hospital dispense almost all of the prescriptions for the patient population.

The elements for Maronde's system of drug use review are (1) a set of standards or definitions of appropriate drug use related to diagnosis; (2) an electronic data processing system permitting on-line retrieval of any patient's drug history for the past six months; and (3) the incorporation of specially trained pharmacists at the terminal site in the clinic to interpret drug-related data and to consult with physicians on prescribing practices. Maronde employed a committee of physicians and pharmacists, with consultation from specialists, to prepare "definitions for drug usage." Besides determining appropriate drug therapy by diagnosis, the committee also dealt with minimum and maximum daily dosage, desired duration of therapy, minimum and maximum quantity limits by prescription order and a maximum limit of the drug which should be in the hands of the patient at any one time. These limits represent the parameters by which exceptional drug use was detected and dealt with.

Even though the formulary in use at LAC-USC limited the drugs in use to 1400, the data to be handled were enormous. Maronde's system, when it became operational, was able to recover stored descriptive information on drugs on a cathode ray tube terminal in the clinic. Its most important use in the clinic was to permit input and access to patient drug history files. A six-month drug history was available for recall while the patient was being treated. Patterns of drug therapy and potential interactions could be readily discerned. New prescription orders were entered directly into the patient's computer record and were transmitted to the pharmacy for dispensing. The key person in the implementation of the drug use review system was the pharmacist, placed in the clinic setting to deal with physicians and nurses at the point drug therapy decisions were made. The pharmacists employed were either graduate pharmacists who had been given a year of specialized training in a clinic, or were recent graduates of the USC School of Pharmacy who receive such experience routinely. It was their responsibility to translate medical diagnoses into computer terminology, to call up and evaluate the patient drug history in relationship to the current prescribed drug therapy, and to recommend necessary alterations to the physician as required.

In addition to the prospective review of prescribing, retrospective analyses of the prescribing patterns of physicians were undertaken using the definitions for drug usage as criteria. These analyses detected (1) excessive drug quantities by individual prescription order, (2) excessive frequency of prescription orders for the same drug for the same patient, and (3) inappropriate concurrent prescribing of drugs which may interact harmfully.

Many inappropriate prescriptions were found, over half being accounted for by fewer than three per cent of the prescribing physicians. A detailed evaluation of the success of the project is not found in the monograph. The system detected many cases of prescribing which fell outside of defined limits. In dollar terms, Maronde estimates that drug costs were cut by 15 per cent as a result of drug use review. The availability of reasonably complete patient drug histories minimized the possibility of inappropriate concurrent prescribing. However, the cost was high, and a subsequent loss of federal funding has ended the availability of on-line prospective review.

References, 0. *Key words:* Formularies.

MARONDE, ROBERT F. Social Security Administration. Office of Research and Statistics, Staff Paper No. 13. DHEW Publication No. (SSA) 73-11853. Washington, D.C., United States Government Printing Office, May 1972.

The Role of Computers in Drug Utilization Review

201 Drug utilization review programs are designed to control the improper use of insurance benefits and inappropriate prescribing practices. Computer processing and communications techniques can be applied to some drug utilization problems, for example, recording and comparing for each of a group of physicians the frequency of prescription orders for generic drugs and for therapeutically-equivalent but more expensive brand name drugs. The compilation of profile data from health records to support empirical standards for drug utilization is seen as less useful than developing standards in terms of patient and situational factors. Computers can assist in record keeping and monitoring functions. Review procedures can be retrospective, prospective, or concurrent. Computer processing of prescription requests and drug histories will be more helpful to patients under prospective or concurrent review systems. Feedback on findings of drug review programs in terms of drug utilization and insurance data should be provided to all practitioners and professional schools. Computer usage can overcome traditional delays in providing this information. A potential problem with computer assistance is maintaining the confidentiality of prescription records. Steps should be taken to minimize improper disclosure.

References, 8. *Key words:* Substitution.

RUCKER, T. DONALD. *American Journal of Hospital Pharmacy* 29 (2):128–134, February 1972.

Drug Utilization and Peer Review in San Joaquin

238 The drug utilization review program of the San Joaquin Foundation for Medical Care and PAID Prescriptions in California uses computerized drug records and a pharmacist-physician committee to control drug utilization and costs in a four-county Medi-Cal program. Automatic monitoring of drug claims reports yields information on duplicate claims (reduced under this program from 10 per cent to less than 0.1 per cent), prescriptions refilled too soon, inappropriate quantities dispensed, inappropriate prescribing by therapeutic class of drug, and patients who receive too many prescriptions in a fixed time period. Examples of patient and physician profiles and pharmacy control reports, are offered.

A committee of four pharmacists and one physician reviews data and challenges unusual physician or pharmacist practices with a letter, which includes the 6-month drug history of the patient involved. This communication and feedback mechanism has been an "outstanding success" and has led to a 12.1 per cent cost savings in the first year from the correction of wasteful practices. Of 60 cases studied, 17 showed marked changes in prescribing and dispensing patterns, resulting in an average annual estimated saving of $18.52 per patient. Drug costs and utilization in the San Joaquin area are considerably below those in the rest of the state. Monitoring patient and physician drug records has also led to a decline in prescribing barbiturates, narcotics and psychotropic drugs. Cases of unnecessary drug therapy are also uncovered.

An educational aspect of the drug utilization review program is the finding and preventing of adverse drug reactions by examining records for potential drug-drug interaction cases. Of the patients studied in a 12-month period, 7.5 per cent were found to have been exposed to potential drug-drug interactions. Adverse drug reactions account for 4–7 per cent of all hospital admissions and may cost up to $2.25 billion annually; 70–80 per cent are avoidable. A program to control the prescribing of excessive quantities (identified from computer records) reduced drug costs by 10 per cent.

References, 12.

TALLEY, ROBERT B.; and LAVENTURIER, MARC F. Presented before the American Association of Foundations for Medical Care, Sea Island, Georgia, August 28, 1972.

1971

A Study of Prescribing Patterns

151

Outpatient prescriptions for seventy-eight prescribed drugs at the Los Angeles County—University of Southern California Medical Center were analyzed to indicate the nature and frequency of inappropriate or undesirable prescribing. The three types of undesirable prescriptions studied were: (1) excessive drug quantities specified in the individual prescriptions; (2) undesirably frequent prescriptions for the same drug; and (3) inappropriate concurrent prescriptions for different drugs.

The definition and criteria of undesirable or inappropriate prescribing were developed by a group of five physicians and two pharmacists for each drug item in the Medical Center formulary for outpatient use. The seventy-eight drugs selected for review represented more than eighty per cent of all outpatient prescriptions dispensed at the Medical Center. A total of 52,733 consecutive prescriptions for the 78 drugs, dispensed over a two and a half month period, were analyzed. No attempt was made to determine if inadequate amounts of drug were prescribed.

Analysis of the data indicated: (1) 13 per cent of the prescriptions called for drug amounts in what were defined as excess quantities. Prescriptions for sedatives and tranquilizers were proportionally high in this category of undesirable prescriptions. Approximately 50 per cent of all prescriptions for excessive quantities were written by thirty physicians (3.4 per cent of the total number of prescribing physicians). Generally, a physician who wrote prescriptions for excessive quantities for one drug wrote excessive quantity prescriptions for other drugs. (2) Only 1.7 per cent of all prescriptions involved undesirably frequent prescriptions of the same drug for a particular patient.

Some outpatients, however, were receiving as many as fifty-four prescriptions over a 112-day period. (3) Many cases were found to be concurrent prescriptions of two different drug products which could result in adverse effects due to drug interaction or drug potentiation. Prescriptions for tranquilizers and sedatives were most frequently involved. Of the total prescriptions, 3.7 per cent were categorized as inappropriate concurrent prescriptions, with each two concurrent prescriptions considered as one event. Generally this type of undesirable prescribing involved an individual receiving prescriptions from two or more physicians.

It was not known whether the physician was aware of other medications currently being taken by the patient, or if each concurrent prescription was actually being taken. A computer system to apprise the physician of a patient's drug record and the suggested prescription quantity is now under development at the Medical Center. The physician would retain the responsibility, however, for making the final prescribing decision.

References, 31.

MARONDE, ROBERT F.; LEE, PETER V.; McCARRON, MARGARET M.; and SEIBERT, STANLEY. *Medical Care* 9 (5):383-395, September-October 1971.

Basic Methods for Optimizing the Rational Prescribing of Psychoactive Drugs

190 Effective prescribing of psychoactive drugs (or of drug products in general) depends on (1) a national computer-assisted drug information network and data bank to record prescription orders and cope with third-party insurance claims, (2) systematic drug utilization review programs to evaluate prescription drug records for conformity to scientific standards for rational prescribing, dispensing and use (perhaps including cost considerations in addition to therapeutic considerations), and (3) a coordinated, systemic, objective information and education service ("a compendium system") for health care professionals.

Standards for rational prescribing should deal with factors such as (1) minimum and maximum drug quantities, appropriate dosages and strengths, refills and adverse reactions, (2) criteria for no drug therapy or delayed drug therapy, (3) relationship of patient condition, age and sex to drug prescribing. With psychoactive drugs, preparation of standards is difficult because guidelines for their efficacy are not yet available, standards for appropriate diagnosis must be developed and a concurrent review information system must be employed (while the patient is being examined) for feedback on therapeutic histories and standards.

To counteract inappropriate prescribing and differences in prescribing habits, a compendium system, like drug utilization review, would be useful and should include a comprehensive reference work on all drug products marketed in the United States, selected information sources by therapeutic category or drug product, and an educational component (perhaps a committee to inform physicians about rational prescribing of specific products). These techniques could save more than $1 billion annually. However, certain marketing practices must be discontinued if unbiased and comprehensive information on drug therapy is to be provided.

References, 6.

RUCKER, T. DONALD. *Journal of Drug Issues 1* (3):326-332, Fall 1971.

1970

Drug Utilization and Drug Utilization Review and Control

30

Drug utilization is defined as "prescribing, dispensing, administering and ingesting" prescription drugs, and effective control of drug utilization is recommended through: public education programs of the Public Health Service; cooperative efforts of the American Medical Association and the American Pharmaceutical Association in discussing drug utilization review and control; concern about drug utilization on the part of the pharmaceutical industry and the development of new approaches to marketing; a national center for collecting, analyzing and disseminating statistics about drug utilization; the establishment of broad policies, priorities, guidelines and liaisons among federal agencies concerned with drug utilization.

The review discusses patterns of drug utilization in the United States, factors influencing drug utilization (such as age, sex, lifestyle), mechanisms of control in the private and public sectors, automated control systems and areas needing additional research.

References, 72.

BRODIE, DONALD C. Public Health Service. Health Services and Mental Health Administration. DHEW Publication No. (HSM) 72-3002. Washington, D.C., United States Government Printing Office, April 1970.

Medi-Cal: California Medicaid: A Management and Utilization Study

38

A 1968-1969 study of management information systems and computerized utilization review techniques showed the potential for significant savings in the administration of public medical assistance programs. The State Department of Health Care Services and the National Pharmaceutical Council, in cooperation with the San Joaquin Foundation for Medical Care and the University of California School of Pharmacy, concluded that: (1) peer review committees can contribute significantly to the improvement of medical care and control of medical care costs; (2) an efficient computerized utilization review system supporting active peer review is effective in achieving significant savings; (3) computerized claims processing can help prevent duplicate payments for services; and (4) computer programs and management techniques can be adapted to medical assistance programs in other states.

The study recommends establishing peer review committees, undertaking a comprehensive analysis of administrative costs, assigning a permanent and unique identification number to each eligible Medicaid person and administering the entire program through the same fiscal agency. It notes that utilization review programs (both prospective and retrospective) should establish norms of service such as: was the service provided needed, was it appropriate to the need, was it of high quality, was it properly priced, and was it provided on a timely basis?

References, 0.

CALIFORNIA DEPARTMENT OF HEALTH CARE SERVICES. Sacramento, The Department, 1970.

No Date

Drug Utilization of a Four Year Cohort of Health Education and Welfare—Neighborhood Health Center Program Participants

112 A drug utilization study of 828 medically indigent persons over the period 1969–1972 under the Kaiser-Permanente program in Oregon showed the following: (1) there was no appreciable change in per capita drug utilization; (2) about 40 per cent of the people received no prescriptions during any year; (3) no more than 8 per cent received an average of more than one prescription per month; (4) per capita prescription expenditures increased. This was explained by an increase in average prescription charge (especially for the 20 most frequently prescribed drugs over the four years) and not by any increase in the number of prescriptions received. From this finding, it was difficult to assess the cost impact of changes in prescription quantities. The report does suggest that increase in dosage unit charges contributed to the increased prescription expenditures. (5) The 25 most frequently prescribed drugs each year accounted for one third of all prescriptions, although these 25 drugs varied each year (for example, of the 25 most frequently prescribed in 1969, only eight were included in 1972); (6) analgesics, anti-infectives, tranquilizers and antitussives accounted for 54 per cent of the prescriptions in any year, and the number of prescriptions received for these categories (except for tranquilizers) as well as average prescription charges increased each year.

The results suggest that drug use review should concentrate on changes in specific drugs prescribed over a period of time, especially by therapeutic class. Pharmacy charges should be periodically reviewed, as should the records of those persons who consistently receive large numbers of prescriptions.

References, 0.

JOHNSON, RICHARD E.; CAMPBELL, WILLIAM H.; AZEVEDO, DANIEL J.; and DRICHAS, MARILYN W. Portland, Oregon, Kaiser Foundation Hospitals, no date.

1970–71 Report on Administration of the Medi-Cal Drug Program for the San Joaquin Foundation for Medical Care on a Prepayment Basis

171 PAID Prescriptions administered the drug portion of the Medi-Cal program for the San Joaquin Foundation for Medical Care, beginning in August 1970 for 43,000–50,000 beneficiaries from 4 counties. It introduced automated drug claims processing and multidisciplinary peer review, yielding cost savings of approximately 10 per cent. PAID Prescriptions received a fixed fee based on population within each aid category. The program is described and analyzed after one year of operation.

About 46 per cent of total drug expenditures were under old age assistance programs. Prescriber analysis revealed 49 of 327 physicians who wrote an unusually high number of prescriptions, and the therapeutic categories of the most frequently prescribed drugs. A similar analysis was performed for 47 of 112 pharmacies considered exceptional; this information is of interest for utilization review.

Price and frequency of prescription data generated under the PAID Prescriptions system were compared for the period before and after fee restrictions were imposed on pharmacies. It was found, for example, that three cough preparations were replaced by three other lower-cost cough preparations. Drug utilization review involved a peer review committee of four pharmacists and one physician that met monthly. The committee disseminates information on usage patterns, recommends voluntary controls and improved prescribing and dispensing procedures, and deals with specific abuses. It examines computer-generated patient profiles considered exceptional on the basis of stated criteria (for example, insufficient quantity of a drug prescribed, or duplicate prescriptions dispensed).

References 0.

PAID PRESCRIPTIONS. San Mateo, California, PAID Prescriptions, no date.

Cross-References

The following abstracts also include information on drug use review:

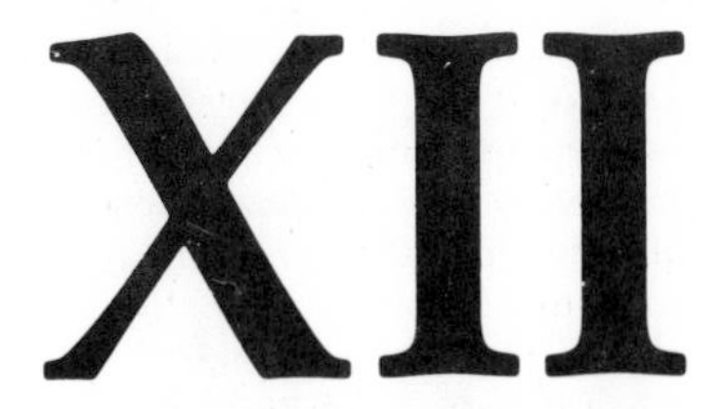

XII
Prescribing Controls: Formulary Restrictions

A formulary is a list of drugs paid for by the program. In addition to limiting the number of drugs available to prescribers, other controls, such as dosage and quantity limits, may be added to further affect prescribing.
Key word: Formularies.

1977

Psychotropic and Analgesic Drug Prescriptions for Patients Seeing Multiple Physicians in a Medicaid Program

225

Drug prescription data were compared for two six-month periods, one before and one after the adoption of a formulary for the Mississippi Medicaid program. Data were selected from a stratified random sample of Mississippi pharmacies. Some findings were: (1) for all drug categories, there was little change in the proportion of patients receiving prescriptions from multiple doctors, (2) for patients receiving both psychotropic and analgesic drugs, nearly 40 per cent of patients in the first period and no patients in the second period received prescriptions from two or more physicians, and (3) patients who received prescriptions from multiple physicians received more total prescriptions than the relative numbers of patients would predict.

References, 1.

SMITH, MICKEY C. *Medical Marketing and Media 12* (*1*):26, 28, 30–31, 34, January 1977.

1976

Will Maximum Allowable Cost Cut Prescription Costs? Let's Take a Good Look!

40

Note: The title of this article misrepresents its content.
Costs for psychotherapeutic drugs at 20 Mississippi pharmacies differed little for formulary (major tranquilizer) and nonformulary (minor tranquilizer) products, yet the impact on patient care was considerable. In an effort to cut

drug costs in the state Medicaid program, which introduced a drug benefit July 1, 1970, a formulary was adopted which excluded minor tranquilizers prescribed by almost every physician. Data on Medicaid prescriptions at 20 randomly selected pharmacies for two 6-month periods (one before and one after the introduction of the formulary—dates unspecified) were compiled for computer analysis. Fifty physicians were interviewed; 60 per cent "went along" with the formulary.

Of more than 100,000 prescriptions, about 9000 were for psychotherapeutic drugs. The cost of these drugs during the second 6-month period was $24,343; cost to Medicaid had minor tranquilizers been prescribed was $24,570. Out-of-pocket costs to Medicaid patients for minor tranquilizers not included in the formulary was $73,080. Extrapolating statewide, savings for 6 months by prescribing psychotherapeutic substitutes from the formulary for minor tranquilizers was only $6,810.

The savings was considered small because prescriptions for major tranquilizers, psychostimulants, combinations and barbiturates increased greatly; these were more costly than minor tranquilizers. Dangers to the patients of prescribing the former drugs are potentially more serious side effects, inappropriateness (drugs not therapeutically equivalent to minor tranquilizers), excessive medication (where only a minor tranquilizer is needed), and the problem of physicians who prescribe minor tranquilizers which Medicaid patients cannot afford (thereby failing to receive drug therapy). The advantages, in terms of quality of patient care, for extending drug benefits to minor tranquilizers seems to outweight the small savings. Cost-benefit judgements about a formulary must consider both economic and therapeutic criteria.

References, 0.

CARLOVA, JOHN. *Drug Topics 120* (4):39–40, February 15, 1976.

Hospital Formularies: Organizational Aspects and Supplementary Components

203 An examination of the nature of supplementary sections and organizational features of hospital formularies suggests that the formulary is not generally employed effectively to transmit drug information and regulations.

Documents used to guide or restrict prescribing and responses to a brief questionnaire were received in February-March 1976 from 44 teaching hospitals with at least 500 beds (out of a national sample of 164 hospitals contacted). Considering that provision of therapeutic guidelines has long been recognized as a supplementary formulary function, it is disappointing that 18 per cent of the formularies were just drug lists. Almost another 22 per cent had few supporting sections. Slightly over half listed drug products both alphabetically and by pharmacologic-therapeutic classification. The principle of generic nomenclature was followed exclusively by 60 per cent and in mixed form by 20 per cent.

Although 80 per cent included a background section on formulary development and use, clear definitions of purpose or other significant information often seemed lacking. Forty per cent had not been recently revised. A little over half the sample formularies devoted sections to prescribing regulations and technical aids of various kinds. The same percentage had provisions more or less effectively aimed at lowering drug costs. Other types of supporting sections, appearing in smaller numbers of formularies, included information on pharmacy services, drug products, patient medical condition and hospital regulations. There was a marked lack of uniformity in physical characteristics. Only about a third were conveniently portable or easily updated. Though nearly half had superior readability, many suffered from small type, weak impression, or other format problems.

General patterns emerging from the study were frequent inconsistency in scope of coverage and in numerous administrative aspects. It is unclear what led to abbreviated guidelines, but it is unlikely that other methods of controlling prescribing or total practitioner knowledge explain the variability.

References, 5.

RUCKER, T. DONALD; and VISCONTI, JAMES A. *American Journal of Hospital Pharmacy 33* (9):912–917, September 1976.

The Massachusetts Drug Formulary Act

245

The provisions of the 1970 Massachusetts Drug Formulary Act, if applied by pharmacies to support generic prescribing and a bid system for the purchase of drug products, will result in savings for pharmacists and consumers, as well as improved inventory control. The Act (included as Appendix A of this paper) requires physicians to include generic or chemical names when prescribing drugs by brand name and creates a commission to develop a formulary of therapeutically equivalent generic substitutes for commonly prescribed brand name drugs. Before the Act was passed, pharmacists were required to dispense the drug product specified. With generic prescribing, however, the pharmacist can dispense equivalent drugs from any manufacturer. If a prescription does not specify generic name as well as brand name, pharmacists must contact the physician and request it.

Limitations of the Act are (1) the formulary covers only a limited number of drug products, so pharmacists cannot dispense chemically equivalent drugs that are not listed, (2) physicians may indicate "no substitute" or "brand only" and thus not allow the pharmacist to substitute drug products, (3) there is no enforcement or penalty provision for physicians who do not include generic names when prescribing by brand name and pharmacists will not always contact physicians to obtain this information.

Compliance in 1972 was estimated at greater than 10 per cent. If pharmacists actively employed the guidelines of the Act, they could reduce inventory and costs. Since pharmacists have the authority to substitute equivalent drug products under generic prescribing, they do not have to maintain inventories of several brands of a product. By requesting bids from manufacturers, selecting the best brand (in terms of equivalency and price) and purchasing that brand in a greater quantity, the pharmacy can guarantee a certain market for the manufacturer (perhaps allowing for reduced manufacturing costs) and obtain the product at a reduced unit cost. A sample form for requesting bids is provided. Thus, if guidelines of the Act are followed, savings on drug costs will result.

References, 5.

TAUBMAN, ALBERT H.; and GOSSELIN, RAYMOND A. *Journal of the American Pharmaceutical Association NS16* (2):71–73, February 1976.

1975

Future of Drug Compendia

60

Five areas relating to drug compendia are discussed: (1) the need for compendia, (2) gaps in compendia, (3) adequacy of compendia specifications, (4) future developments for compendia, and (5) the critique of the official compendia by the Drug Bioequivalence Study Panel of the Office of Technology Assessment (OTA).

Specifically, the following points are elaborated upon: (1) the standards establishing role of the compendia, (2) the need for the development of additional test procedures and for the broader application of established procedures, (3) theoretical differences between various tests and the statistical requirements for their performance, including the difference between testing for unit-to-unit variation within a single lot and testing for inter-lot variations, and (4) criticisms raised by the OTA report. The implications of the OTA report viewed as a consumer-oriented reaction are discussed. The fact that no person with expertise on the official compendia was included on the OTA panel is emphasized.

Future developments anticipated are for (1) the control over the suitability of drug dosage form delivery systems, (2) additional specifications relating to in vitro tests which serve to indicate in vivo performance, and (3) increased emphasis on the dissemination of background information relating to the adoption of a given procedure or specification, including information on why the specified procedure was adopted over other known procedures.

References, 0.

FELDMANN, EDWARD G. *Journal of the American Pharmaceutical Association NS15* (4):198–201, April 1975.

How Drugs Attain Formulary Listing

186

Representing various regions and sizes, 305 hospitals receiving Medicare funds were surveyed by questionnaire to determine formulary use (required by Medicare law) and the selection process for drugs included in the formulary. The number of hospitals returning the questionnaires was 172, or 56 per cent.

Despite Medicare requirements, 18 per cent of the hospitals did not have a formulary. The responses of the 141 hospitals that did have a formulary or drug list were analyzed by bed size (8 groups from 6–24 beds to 500 and more beds). Of the hospitals analyzed, 73 per cent operated with a formulary system—a formal selection and evaluation process; therefore, up to 27 per cent of the hospitals may include drugs in the formulary with no evaluation. A pharmacy and therapeutics committee approved the formulary in 89 per cent of the hospitals. The committee usually has full responsibility for evaluating drugs considered for inclusion in the formulary. Written policies for approving drug inclusion in the formulary were found in 65 per cent of the hospitals. The amount of information required from physicians who request the inclusion of a drug in the formulary increases with hospital size. Most hospitals allow physicians to prescribe drugs which are not in the formulary. The number of factors used in evaluating drugs for inclusion increases with hospital size. Most hospitals revise their formularies one or more times a year.

The data support the thesis that hospitals act effectively in selecting drugs for inclusion in formularies. Guidelines are suggested, such as establishing procedures for obtaining permission to use drugs not in the formulary, specifying information to be obtained in evaluating drugs and indicating the information to be included in the formulary on each drug.

References, 4.

ROLANDS, THOMAS F.; and WILLIAMS, ROBERT B. *Hospitals 49* (2):87–89, January 16, 1975.

Drug Usage Review and Inventory Analysis in Promoting Rational Parenteral Cephalosporin Therapy

220

The pharmacy and therapeutics committee of the Shands Teaching Hospital at the University of Florida formed a subcommittee to evaluate parenteral cephalosporins on the basis of inventory, cost and use data. The subcommittee rejected a request to add cephapirin to the hospitals's formulary because budgetary constraints precluded adding a drug offering no significant advantages. It determined that cefazolin, which the subcommittee felt was preferred in most cases, and cephalothin, with which the medical staff had more experience, were the main drugs to be considered. It also agreed that cephalosporins were being overused for staphylococcal infections.

The pharmacy supplied data on expenditures for top dollar usage systemic antibiotics in 1973 and 1974; a comparison of costs of cephalothin, cefazolin and cephapirin at different dosage regimens; and a classification of cephalothin and cefazolin orders. Relative costs varied with the dosage schedule used. The subcommittee concluded that cefazolin was often used in too high a dose (1 g rather than 500 mg) and at too frequent intervals (q 6 hr rather than q 8 hr) and that modifying this would be the most economical approach. Data and recommendations were presented to the full committee, which notified the medical staff by memorandum that it would delete cephalothin from the formulary in 6 weeks. A decision to purchase cefazolin on bid lowered the price further.

Objections by some staff members and pharmaceutical company representatives brought the cephalosporin decision up for debate again. Review of the pharmacology of both drugs turned up articles suggesting that cephalothin may be less nephrotoxic and that it penetrates the eye. The committee modified its decision slightly to permit its use in ophthalmologic and impaired renal function patients. Usage of cefazolin increased dramatically thereafter, and dosage regimens changed somewhat. Continual education has proven necessary, however. Factors that will have to be monitored in the future include substitution of other antibiotics, trends in route of administration and related side effets, optimum storage possibilities, drug shortages and changes in patient population.

References, 12. *Key words:* Drug utilization review.

SIMON, WAYNE A.; THOMPSON, LOUIS; CAMPBELL, STUART; and LANTOS, ROBERT L. *American Journal of Hospital Pharmacy 32* (*11*):1116–1121, November 1975.

Prescribing Patterns, Physician Reactions, and Economic Effects of Closed and Open Formularies

224 The attitudes of a random sample of Mississippi physicians to the change from an open to a closed formulary are reported and preliminary results of an analysis of more than 100,000 Medicaid prescriptions dispensed by 20 pharmacies in a 6-month period under the 2 types of formularies are summarized.

In the semistructured interview of physicians, with regard to their prescribing patterns, patient interaction and opinions on the Medicaid program, more than half reported that they attempted to prescribe drugs covered by the formulary. Approximately 20 per cent indicated a greater cost consciousness on the part of Medicaid patients, who asked the physician to prescribe from the formulary. Two-thirds of the physicians said they attempted to comply. When drugs were removed from the formulary (and the full cost had to be borne by the patient), 70 per cent of the physicians continued to prescribe such drugs. More than 80 per cent did not believe that formulary restrictions applied to hospital drug orders.

If a drug is deleted from the formulary, third-party program expenditures for it will decline, but more costly and less appropriate drugs may be substituted. Therefore, social costs must be considered in the removal of drugs from a formulary. It is suggested that efforts to improve prescribing be made through utilization review programs, not through local closed formulary programs.

References, 0. *Key words:* Drug utilization review.

SMITH, MICKEY C. *In* Anonymous. *Revolution in Health Care.* Proceedings of a Symposium Held in Columbia, South Carolina, September 30, 1974. Nutley, New Jersey, Hoffmann-LaRoche, Incorporated, 1975. Pages 40–45.

Effects of Closing a Medicaid Formulary on Prescribing Psychotherapeutic Drugs

229 A closed formulary, adopted September 1, 1971 by the Mississippi Medicaid Drug Program, did not include minor tranquilizers. Physicians could: (1) continue to prescribe minor tranquilizers, forcing these patients to pay for the prescriptions themselves (or failing to have the prescriptions filled because of the cost); (2) prescribe the one minor tranquilizer inexplicably retained in the formulary (which none of them did); (3) prescribe a replacement drug (a major tranquilizer or other psychotherapeutic drug); or (4) discontinue therapy.

Data were collected from a random sample of 20 Mississippi pharmacies for January 1 to June 30, 1971, and January 1 to June 20, 1972. Of more than 100,000 prescriptions, 9000 were for psychotherapeutic drugs.

Prescribing frequency for all drugs increased by 11 per cent after the closed formulary was instituted. Significant increases were found in prescription volume for all psychotherapeutic drugs remaining in the formulary (major tranquilizers, psychostimulants, combinations, barbiturates), but in many cases of replacement for minor tranquilizers, lower doses were prescribed. Of all psychotherapeutic prescriptions written in the closed formulary period, 38 per cent were for minor tranquilizers not listed in the formulary and dispensed outside the Medicaid program. Prescribing habits of a sample of 16 physicians are discussed.

Medicaid costs for psychotherapeutic drugs in the formulary for the 1972 period dispensed by the pharmacies studied were $24,343. Had minor tranquilizers been included, costs were calculated at $24,570, extrapolating to an average annual statewide savings of $13,620 (0.01 per cent of the total Medicaid budget). It was also estimated that this saving to the Medicaid Commission caused the people it is serving to incur additional personal drug costs of $73,080. Implications for quality of patient care are examined, and the effectiveness of other psychotherapeutic drugs as replacements for minor tranquilizers is questioned.

References, 14.

SMITH, MICKEY C.; and ROWLAND, CLAYTON R. Department of Health Care Administration. University, Mississippi, University of Mississippi, no date (1975?).

Potential Economic Effects of a Brand Standardization Policy in a 1000-Bed Hospital

237

The potential economic effects of a brand standardization policy in a 1000-bed hospital utilizing a unit dose drug distribution system were examined. Fifty commercially available, high-use, nonproprietary drugs were selected for study and their drug usage and drug inventory costs were compared under a formulary and nonformulary system.

Drug usage cost was defined as the dollar value expended by the hospital in order to purchase drugs administered, and drug inventory cost was defined as the dollar value of drug products being stored for use in the hospital pharmacy. For the fifty drugs under examination, the use of this brand standardization policy was found to yield potential savings of more than $35,000 for drug usage costs and in excess of $9,000 for drug inventory costs. As a result of this study, it was concluded that a brand standardization policy would lower drug usage and inventory costs, that it would reduce the quantity of inventory items, and that such a policy could be implemented with minimal difficulty.

References, 20.

SWIFT, ROBERT G.; and RYAN, MICHAEL R. *American Journal of Hospital Pharmacy* 32 (12):1242–1250, December 1975.

1974

Some Legal Aspects of the Hospital Formulary System

63

The article discusses various ways to obtain consent between the physician and hospital (in particular, the hospital pharmacy) such that a brand name drug prescription can be filled with its generic substitute contained in the approved hospital formulary. The two methods discussed are: (1) prior general consent, which is given prior to the writing of a particular prescription and applies to all medication orders unless otherwise indicated, and (2) current consent, which is indicated at the time of issuing a prescription. Various imprints on a prescription order form to indicate current consent are mentioned. The practice of using prior general consent is no longer recommended and hospitals are urged to adopt a method of current consent. Differences with respect to expressing consent between the 1960 and 1964 versions of the Statement of Guiding Principles on the Operation of the Hospital Formulary System are extensively discussed. Other legal issues in the operation of a formulary system discussed are the labeling of containers and the relationship of the Federal Trade Commission to the system.

References, 43. *Key words:* Inpatient settings.

FINK, JOSEPH L. III. *American Journal of Hospital Pharmacy 31 (1)*:86–90, January 1974.

Providing Quality Drugs Economically. The Role of State Formularies

157 The Tennessee Medicaid Drug Program is attempting to control costs by combining an "open-controlled" formulary with utilization review and bioequivalency evaluation. Before adopting the program, a survey was made of relevant studies and other states' experiences.

Formularies have been used to cut costs by decreasing inventories and recommending cheaper products. They are also convenient for data processing and peer review. On the other hand, they may restrict choice of therapy, require frequent revision and have administrative costs. Some simply list all agents by generic name to facilitate coding; others may restrict drugs, sources or both. Medical and economic judgement is involved and risk-benefit ratios must be weighed. Savings of up to $40 million a year from generic prescribing have been projected. However, the significance of inequivalent bioavailability of chemically equivalent products is controversial. Several recent studies question the availability of sufficient information for pharmacists to objectively evaluate competing products.

States that have tried formularies that significantly restrict reimbursable drugs have not achieved the expected savings. Not enough is known yet about those states that are attempting to encourage generic prescribing, though a Massachusetts survey suggests that these efforts have been largely ineffective in altering prescribing habits. Several reports have indicated that programs which carefully monitor claims for abuses have cut costs significantly. Utilization surveillance with peer review may cut medical as well as drug costs by improving therapy.

Based on the available data, Tennessee decided to build into its program a relatively nonrestrictive formulary, a systematic review system and efforts to evaluate relative product efficacy. The formulary encompasses most prescribed drugs, with exceptions like OTC or anorectic drugs except in specified conditions. Price ceilings have been set for some dozen drugs at a calculated savings of over $400,000 a year. A contract was made with the University of Tennessee College of Pharmacy for a bioavailability testing program for certain drugs and eventually the formulary will include source limitations. Routine checks are made on drug utilization records for potential abuse by patients, prescribers or pharmacists. There are also renewal restrictions on all drugs. The program seems to be working efficiently; the 1973 cost per claim was only $4.29, professional fee included. It should also contribute important information on the significance of bioavailability problems.

References, 34. *Key words:* Drug utilization review.

MEYER, MARVIN C.; BATES, HERBERT, JR.; and SWIFT, ROBERT G. *Journal of the American Pharmaceutical Association NS14* (*12*):663–666, December 1974.

Physician Acceptance of Three Proposed Programs Designed to Reduce Prescription Prices

165

Physicians' perception of prescription drug prices as excessive was found to be significantly related to receptivity to methods of reducing prescription drug prices by repeal of state antisubstitution laws, the use of a federal or a community formulary, and to a willingness to accept product selection by pharmacists if consumer price savings were assured.

A random sample of 500 physicians received a pretested mail questionnaire on university letterhead; the response rate was 64.6 per cent. On physicians' attitudes toward the average price paid by consumers for prescription drugs, 13.1 per cent believed that prescription drugs were a bargain for the value received, 36.1 per cent felt that they were priced about right for the value received, and 37.3 per cent thought that they were generally overpriced. Younger physicians and those in institutional practice tended to believe prescription drug prices were excessive. Physicians in large communities and those who were heavy prescribers tended to believe drug prices were about right or a bargain. Of those who believed drugs were overpriced, 51.5 per cent blamed drug manufacturers, 38.1 per cent blamed pharmacists, and none blamed the prescribers themselves for excessive drug prices.

Earlier research is cited in which three-fourths of the private physicians surveyed said they considered prices when prescribing, but few could accurately estimate (within 20 per cent) the prices of their chosen drugs; estimates were consistently low. On the question of the acceptance of pharmacists substituting less expensive chemically equivalent prescription drugs, 57.3 per cent indicated high acceptance; of those who believed prices were excessive, 76.3 per cent indicated high acceptance. On their attitude toward a federal formulary, 25 per cent indicated acceptance; of those who believed prices were excessive, 37.5 per cent indicated acceptance. On attitudes toward a community formulary, 32.1 per cent indicated acceptance; of those who believed prices were excessive, 43.0 per cent indicated acceptance. On attitudes toward repeal of antisubstitution laws, 27.6 per cent were in favor; of those who believed prices were excessive, 40.6 per cent were in favor. Efforts should be made to provide price information to physicians.

References, 23. *Key words:* Maximum allowable cost.

NELSON, ARTHUR A.; and GAGNON, JEAN P. *Drugs in Health Care 1* (*1*):27–37, Summer 1974.

1973

The Formulary in Your Future

8

With the establishment of formularies, the traditional privilege of the physician to prescribe according to his own judgment is being threatened. This article traces the development of the drug formulary, discusses its present role and the role of the physician in the whole scheme. Nonhospital formularies presently exist in at least six states and the one in Massachusetts is cited as a case in point. A formulary in Maryland is the newest addition to the roster. It is an attempt to save consumers' money, but physician reaction has not been positive.

Other states are involved in the creation of formularies, despite the fact that only a small percentage of physicians have endorsed the concept. The ultimate outcome will probably be the establishment of a federal formulary tied in with a national health insurance plan. Despite physicians' arguments that they prescribe a drug that they believe will be most effective and reasonably priced, the race to create formularies still goes on.

References, 0.

ANONYMOUS: *Physician's Management 13 (10)*:33–34, 40, 42–44, 49, 53, October 1973.

The Restrictive Formulary and Drug Use Review in a Medicare Out-of-Hospital Prescription Drug Program

127

The restrictive formulary and drug use review are discussed in relation to three requirements of an out-of-hospital Medicare drug program: (1) assurance of drug product quality, (2) assurance of the quality of drug use, and (3) cost control.

In a restrictive federal formulary, only the "best available" drug products would presumably be listed, thereby insuring drug quality and lowered drug costs. The role of the Food and Drug Administration (FDA) in assuring drug quality is discussed. In comparison with a restrictive formulary, the FDA is viewed as the better vehicle to assure drug quality for all Americans. The reasons why drug use review is viewed as a better method than the restrictive formulary for preventing inappropriate (over-, under-, or mis-prescribing) drug use are discussed. The necessity to establish criteria for optimal drug use and the level of acceptable variation in advance of review in order to evaluate empirical data is discussed. Drug use review would need to be established and implemented on a local level, with federal and state guidance. The Professional Standards Review Organization system should include a requirement for drug use review. Neither drug use review nor a restrictive formulary are viewed as the appropriate means to control the costs of drug therapy.

References, 11.

KNAPP, DAVID A. *National Association of Retail Druggists Journal 95 (20)*:14–16, October 15, 1973.

Pharmacy Purchasing, Formularies and Prices Paid for Drugs: A Survey of Hospitals in Southern New York State

161

A survey of practices in hospital pharmacies was carried out in the southern counties of New York State, with the cooperation of the American Hospital Service (AHS), in order to see to what extent the concept of "prudent buyer" was pertinent.

Questionnaires were sent by mail to 154 hospitals affiliated with AHS and 125 returned responses. The major aspects discussed were formulary practice, market concentration among pharmaceutical suppliers to hospitals and prices paid by hospitals for drugs. Of the responding hospitals, 88 per cent had implemented the formulary concept and most were kept current. In over half of the hospitals, between 95–100 per cent of all prescriptions were based on formulary drugs; however, on the whole, the formulary had a varied effect on drug choice. There was also variation in the extent to which hospitals relied on any manufacturer as a drug supplier, although leaders were in evidence. Almost all noted a price advantage when dealing with manufacturers rather than wholesalers, in addition to other advantages.

In measuring hospitals as "prudent buyers", hospitals were asked about the purchase of six cited drugs according to brand specified, price paid and frequency of order. While Table 8 shows a wide variation in price as well as in preference for generic vs. trade name drugs, a bias against generic drugs was evident. If generic drugs were tested for biological efficacy and quality, as they are being done in Canada at minimal cost, there could be a greater willingness to purchase generically without fear of loss of quality. Suggestions were also offered to improve the rationality of prescribing and purchasing, such as developing and improving formularies and using alternative drugs.

References, 10. *Key words:* Substitution.

MULLER, CHARLOTTE; and KRASNER, MELVIN. *American Journal of Hospital Pharmacy 30* (9):781–789, September 1973.

An Analysis of the Adequacy of Medicaid Prescriptions

183

Because of the circuitous cause and effect relationship between poverty and ill health and the key role assigned to Medicaid to alleviate this problem, a study was designed to test the adequacy of the Medicaid program in Georgia. Adequacy was defined as the degree to which the 600 drugs on Georgia's Medical Assistance Drug List (MADL) conform to those prescribed for Medicaid patients.

The study was conducted among 41 physicians in a four-county area of northeast Georgia during a 30-day period in the winter of 1971. The physicians were asked to use prenumbered prescription blanks to indicate the number of prescription orders written for Medicaid patients. All local pharmacies were checked to determine the number of prescriptions dispensed for MADL drugs, i.e., those covered for reimbursement. A hypothesis that noncovered drugs exceeded 5 per cent of those prescribed for Medicaid patients, and a null hypothesis that they did not, were considered. When inadequacy was found to be 4.88 per cent in the full sample of 1,477 prescriptions dispensed, the null hypothesis "was not accepted because the data gathered indicate that the difference between the observed and theoretical value was statistically significant."

Other analyses show (1) significant correlation between physician specialty and adequacy, with general surgery lowest at 83.78 per cent and ophthalmology, E.E.N.T. and orthopedic surgery highest at 96.67 per cent, and (2) physicians classed as high-volume prescribers (17 or more orders) prescribe more uncovered drugs. Many prenumbered prescription orders (72 or 15.45 per cent) were unlocated, perhaps because many were for noncovered drugs. Adding these to the located Medicaid prescriptions yields 9.23 per cent inadequacy for this class. Conclusions are that the MADL is 95.12 per cent adequate for patients' needs, that physician specialties significantly affect adequacy, and that physicians who prescribe many covered drugs also prescribe the most noncovered ones.

References, 10: *Key words:* Drug utilization review.

RILEY, DAVID A.; BRAUCHER, CHARLES L.; and KOTZAN, JEFFREY A. *Journal of the American Pharmaceutical Association NS13 (10)*:571–573, October 1973.

1972

Insights into Public Assistance Medical Care Expenditures

93

The purpose of the study was to examine the popular belief that states with closed formulary (drug list) systems have lower expenditures for public assistance medical care programs than do states with open or nonrestricted formulary systems. The data analyzed indicate that no relationship exists between the type of formulary system and the medical care expenditures for all states.

The closed and open formulary systems of nine Western and ten Southern states were analyzed and compared. Data on public assistance medical care expenditures were supplied by the United States Department of Health, Education and Welfare for a four-year period (fiscal 1967 through fiscal 1970). Analysis of the data led to two specific findings: (1) states with closed formulary systems spent, in general, more on a per capita basis for total medical care expenditures than did states with no formularies or with open formularies, and (2) Southern states with an open formulary system spent less on drug expenditures per recipient than did Southern states with a closed formulary system; while in Western states, expenditures were slightly more in open formulary states.

The authors discuss the additional costs involved in the operation of a closed formulary system. Such costs include both direct, e.g., administrative, costs and indirect costs, such as the possible increase in total health care expenditures due to the possible nonavailability of the preferred drug in the closed formulary system. The authors conclude with a summary of other studies on peer review and utilization control programs in order to evaluate their efficacy in reducing medical care expenditures. These methods were suggested to be preferable to closed formulary systems in reducing public assistance medical care expenditures.

References, 13.

HAMMEL, ROBERT W. *Journal of the American Medical Association 219 (13)*:1740–1744, March 27, 1972.

Product Selection: Community Formularies and Legal Aspects

118

Dr. Kanig argues that the entire burden of selection of drug products for generic substitution should not be placed onto the pharmacist alone. He advocates a system wherein a formulary is established on a state or national level which contains drug products which were judged to be equivalent by a council of experts, based on their evaluation of relevant clinical and biological data. The pharmacist could substitute generically within the formulary if he desired and would be required to if so requested by the patient.

The view of the pharmacist's role in product selection is thus opposite to that of the American Pharmaceutical Association, which stated in its 1971 "white paper" that ". . . the pharmacist would also assume the responsibility for determining that the substituted product is as effective therapeutically as the one prescribed."

While Dr. Kanig agrees that the pharmacist is indeed the only drug expert on the health care team, he feels that being an expert does not enable one to make judgments on biological equivalence among several drug products allegedly equivalent. The concept of Good Manufacturing Practices, in which all aspects of the procedures used in producing drug products are controlled, and its impact on generic substitution is discussed. The Kentucky formulary system, upon which the advocated model system is based, is described.

References, 0.

KANIG, JOSEPH L. *American Journal of Pharmacy 144* (5):133–138, September–October 1972.

1971

Drug Substitutions

6

This article elucidates the American Medical Association position on the repeal of the antisubstitution law and on hospital formularies. The negative feelings concerning the repeal of this law are not in contradiction of support of hospital formularies. The hospital formulary system does not provide blanket authorization for dispensing a nonproprietary drug or a proprietary drug different from the one prescribed. However, it does allow the physician to use his discretion and professional judgement at the time of prescribing, to approve or disapprove the dispensing of a nonproprietary drug or a proprietary drug other than that prescribed. Opposition to the repeal of the law is based on the premise that blanket delegation of the privilege to substitute would remove the physician's right to exercise his medical judgement. With the implementation of the hospital formulary, this privilege is insured.

References, 0.

ANONYMOUS. *Hospital Formulary Management* 6 (12): 29, December 1971.

The Massachusetts Drug Formulary

152 The Massachusetts Drug Formulary, established by law August 21, 1970, contains an alphabetical list of commonly prescribed brand names, followed by generic names, for single ingredient drugs generally available in Massachusetts. Some over-the-counter items are included for which payment is permitted under the Massachusetts Medical Assistance program. Excluded are sustained-action dosage forms, drugs protected by patent rights, drugs declared ineffective by the FDA and combination drugs under review by the FDA at the time the formulary was being prepared (1970–1971). Physicians will be required to include the generic name when prescribing any brand name drug listed in the formulary. The formulary will be revised periodically.

The HEW Task Force on Prescription Drugs report (February 7, 1969) is cited to support the use of low cost drug equivalents—an estimated saving of 22.5–36.3 per cent had generic drugs been dispensed for 63 brand name products in 1966. The Task Force report and an American Pharmaceutical Association position paper (March 1971) are cited to support the contention of therapeutic or clinical equivalence between generic and brand name drugs.

References, 5. *Key words:* Substitution.

MASSACHUSETTS DEPARTMENT OF PUBLIC HEALTH. *New England Journal of Medicine* 285 (4):232–233, July 22, 1971.

Drug Insurance, Formularies, and Pharmacy

191 The appropriate role of a formulary in a government drug insurance program, and considerations in deciding whether to exclude a particular drug, are discussed in terms of therapeutic, economic and administrative criteria. The function of a formulary might be to ensure that only the best drugs are prescribed. Drugs could be excluded on therapeutic grounds because they are ineffective, combination products without special merit, are of high potential risk, or are less efficacious than another product for the same condition. In the first two cases, it makes more sense for the Food and Drug Administration (FDA) to withdraw the product from the market. Determining restrictions on the use of high risk drugs could also be more efficiently done by the FDA, with insurance programs providing utilization review. A useful formulary role might be to list drugs of superior efficacy. Since scientific evidence is often insufficient to determine relative drug efficacy, however, a list of recommended drugs would seem preferable to a mandatory formulary.

A formulary is often recommended for the purpose of controlling drug costs. It would be wiser to rely on more direct government measures to facilitate competitive pricing, negotiate reasonable prices, or purchase drugs by standard procurement procedures, in order to achieve this purpose. A formulary would be less effective because: physicians often object to restrictions on their prescribing practices for economic reasons; good substitute products often do not exist; a recent Social Security Administration study suggests that formularies may raise inventory costs in hospital pharmacies; and community pharmacies would still have to carry nonformulary products for nongovernment patrons. Administrative considerations entail weighing any potential therapeutic or pricing gains against the costs of administrative mechanisms and the high likelihood that patients, physicians and pharmaceutical manufacturers will circumvent or force alterations in the formulary. The conclusion is that basic therapeutic and economic problems must be provided for in different ways before a formulary can be used as a supplementary tool to help achieve program objectives.

References, 0.

RUCKER, T. DONALD. *Medical Marketing and Media 6 (10)*:11–12, 14, 16–18, October 1971.

Medicaid. Payment of Reasonable Charges for Prescribed Drugs

230

This federally-prepared manual deals with reasonable charges for prescribed drugs and covers the following items: authorization (the law, regulations and other factors); prescription pricing methods and options; variations in reimbursement for prescribed drugs by different types of licensed authorized practitioners; formularies and implementation guidelines.

The federal drug formulary policy states: "The use of a formulary is optional, as are provisions for use of generic drugs. Where either is employed, there must be standards for quality, safety and effectiveness under the supervision of professional personnel." States implementing formularies should consider these guidelines: medications should meet FDA standards for identity, strength, safety, quality, purity and effectiveness; state agencies should strive for economy consistent with these standards; formularies should be flexible and consider professional prerogatives; formulary committees should include physicians, pharmacologists, pharmacists and other professional personnel to revise the formulary periodically; procedures for additions and deletions to the formulary and for the reimbursement of nonlisted items should be formulated; a code number from the FDA National Drug Code Directory should be assigned to each item for ease of electronic data processing. Hospital formularies offer up-to-date information on drugs and drug therapy and are maintained by a staff committee.

The American Society of Hospital Pharmacists' *American Hospital Formulary Service* distributes guidelines for hospitals to use in preparing their formularies. Approximately 20 states in the Medicaid program control drug costs and prescribing standards through the use of a formulary. Some also limit prescribing to generic drugs and establish a price ceiling. Few states can afford comprehensive drug service and usually limit reimbursable drugs to those in a formulary. Some states without formularies exclude classes of drugs such as multivitamins. Drugs may have chemical and proprietary names in addition to generic names; dispensing combination products which contain therapeutic equivalents of substances prescribed by generic name can be difficult.

The successful formulary in Pennsylvania includes 90 per cent of all commonly used drugs and includes price information on which pharmacists base their mark-up. In sum, formularies define payable drugs, simplify prescription auditing and processing as well as drug and price coding, and allow some control over drug prices. However, many physicians will ignore a formulary or see it as interference with professional prerogatives, and formularies may easily become inflexible or outdated.

The appendices present excerpts from Title XIX of the Social Security Act and the *Code of Federal Regulations,* and the Kansas state survey for determination of variable dispensing fees.

References, 0.

SOCIAL AND REHABILITATION SERVICE. MEDICAL SERVICES ADMINISTRATION. DHEW Publication No. SRS-MSA-196-1971. Washington, D.C., United States Government Printing Office, 1971.

1970
A Community Formulary for Delaware?

62

In 1968, the American Pharmaceutical Association recommended the establishment of community formularies as a way of reducing drug costs to patients. Representatives of the medical and pharmaceutical professions in a given community would screen and evaluate drug products for chemical equivalency and therapeutic efficacy in a manner analogous to a pharmacy and therapeutics committee in a hospital. Tasks include: providing a compilation of drugs which, when prescribed, will reduce patient costs while maintaining high quality therapy; advising health professionals in the community of the advantages resulting from the use of a formulary; and promoting cooperation among the health professions. Potential cost savings would result from reducing pharmacy inventories of multiple brands of a given drug product and dispensing only the approved product (if the prescriber so designates), and from purchasing drugs in quantity.

In Delaware, the Formulary Advisory Board is composed of 4 physicians, 3 pharmacists, 1 dentist and 1 osteopathic physician, selected by their professional organizations for three-year terms. In addition, presidents of the professional organizations serve as nonvoting members. The board meets at least once a quarter to evaluate and review proposed additions to, or deletions from, the formulary. The published list provides nonproprietary names, trade names (with cross-references) and manufacturers' names, and is supplied to all physicians, pharmacists and dentists. Prescribers may use formulary or regular prescription blanks, writing "formulary" on the latter if it is desired that the drug be the formulary-approved product.

References, 4.

FINK, JOSEPH L. III. *Delaware Medical Journal 62* (2):41–43, February 1970.

1969

Pharmaceutical Aspects of the Australian National Health Scheme

92

The Australian national health care plan, an extensive scheme for providing medicines in addition to other health care services to its citizenry, is discussed. Pharmaceutical Benefits, available to anyone with a prescription from a certified medical practitioner, represents the most expensive area of health care benefits provided by the government since they are not connected with health insurance and approximately 80 per cent of the medication supplied is paid for under this scheme.

To help standardize the scheme, the Department of Health issues a *Schedule of Pharmaceutical Benefits,* which lists the drugs allowed under coverage and subdivides this list according to those which can be freely supplied, those which are restricted and those which are chemicals for use in extemporaneous preparations. An additional feature of this *Schedule* is that it lists the maximum quantity prescribed at any one time, how often the prescription can be renewed, its price and a code indicating the approved manufacturer. Since calculations and clerical work are complex and tedious, billing and payments have been computerized and systematized so that pharmacists can be paid at the end of each month. Some abuse of the system has occurred, but there has been a minimum of complaints from health care professionals.

While the cost of the program has increased from $15.4 million in 1951 to $104 million in 1967, the United States can still learn many valuable lessons from the Australians in the initiation of plans for third-party payment of prescriptions.

References, 0.

HALL, NATHAN A. *Journal of the American Pharmaceutical Association NS9* (4):184–186, April 1969.

1968

The Drug Prescribers

242

The HEW Task Force on Prescription Drugs investigated: (1) the prescribing patterns of physicians, their training and their information sources on drugs; (2) questions of drug quality (chemical, biological and clinical equivalence, drug standards and quality control); and (3) the use of formularies or drug lists. The various therapeutic judgments that must be made by drug prescribers are described, along with the teaching of pharmacology as a clinical science in several United States medical schools.

The ways in which physicians receive information are examined; for example, medical journals, drug compendia, textbooks, industry advertising, detail men and drug samples. In one study, 57 per cent of 141 physicians indicated that the initial source of information about a new drug was the detail man. In another study, 85 per cent of the physicians reported great confidence in the information provided by detail men.

Various aspects of the drug equivalency controversy are presented. Brand name manufactureres claim to have quality control standards higher than those of low cost generic drug manufacturers. The *United States Pharmacopeia* and the *National Formulary* are described and assessed, and found adequate for their purposes. Responsibilities of the FDA and the Division of Biologic Standards (DBS) are described. The development of various formularies and drug lists are described.

References, 92. *Key words:* Substitution.

TASK FORCE ON PRESCRIPTION DRUGS. Background Papers. Office of the Secretary. United States Department of Health, Education, and Welfare. Washington, D.C., United States Government Printing Office, 1968.

1967

The Formulary System: Product of the Teaching Hospital

69

This article reviews the historical development of formularies and pharmacopeias and discusses the relationship between the two standards. The philosophy of the formulary system is discussed. In the United States, the teaching hospitals led in promoting the formulary system. The history of the formulary is traced from its beginning at the New York Hospital in 1816. The early formularies were developed in order to present a compilation of drugs or drug combinations that were in common use; the formulary was not intended to serve an evaluative or critical function. Selectivity in formulary listings began about 1900. Ten principles upon which the operation of the hospital formulary system should be based are suggested. The role of the pharmacist in promoting the acceptance of the hospital formulary is discussed.

References, 0. *Key words:* Inpatient settings.

FRANCKE, DON E. *Hospitals 41* (22):110, 112, 114, 116, November 16, 1967.

1966

The Financial Effects of Formularies in Hospitals

189

The financial performance of pharmacies in 24 nonteaching Chicago hospitals was assessed through two measures: cost of drugs per inpatient day and the formulary inventory turnover rate. For the size of hospital studied (216–417 bed capacity), the data showed, paradoxically, that as formularies become more restrictive, the financial performance of the pharmacies tends to deteriorate. However, the data also showed that several other factors affect the pharmacy's financial performance: consent agreements, number of items stocked, frequency of trial of new drugs and hospital size. Consent agreements were associated with both an increase in the inventory turnover rate and, especially, with a decrease in drug cost per inpatient day, thus leading to improved financial performance. Financial performance also improved as frequency of trial of new drugs decreased and as hospital size increased.

References, 3.

ROSNER, MARTIN, M. *American Journal of Hospital Pharmacy 23* (12):673–675, December 1966.

1960

The Effect of a Drug Formulary on Costs and Quality of Medical Care in a Public Medical Program

74

The development of a formulary, physician compliance and effects on drug costs and quality of patient care in the Baltimore City Medical Care Program for indigent persons in the 1950's are evaluated. The program is state funded but administered by the city health department. Drug costs were found to affect the financial stability of the program and forced the development of a formulary. Use of the formulary (now up to 70 per cent of all prescriptions) was increased through a program to educate the 300 participating physicians and has reduced the average prescription cost (from $2.03 to $1.90) and stabilized annual per capita drug costs. An advisory committee questions physicians when nonformulary or costly drugs are prescribed; this results in the physicians' "sober evaluation" of therapeutic procedures, often leading to better patient care.

The medical care program covers an initial outpatient physical examination, home and office care by a physician of the patient's choice, outpatient consultation and treatment by specialists, as well as laboratory services at designated hospitals, limited dental care and eyeglasses, drugs and medical supplies; inpatient care is not included. The average number of prescriptions per person was 5.3 and drug expenditures accounted for nearly 37 per cent of the total cost of medical care services. Data are provided on the pharmacist fee schedule (based on wholesale cost of ingredients), costs of various components of the medical care program, prescription numbers and costs (1949–1959) and drug use and costs by classification and formulary status.

References, 1.

FURSTENBERG, FRANK F.; and CLINE, RALEIGH. *In* Tenth Annual Group Health Instutute of Group Health Associations of America. *Proceedings.* Columbus, Ohio, The Institute, May 1960. Pages 167–179.

Cross-References

For further information on formularies, see:

ABSTRACT NUMBER	PAGE NUMBER	ABSTRACT NUMBER	PAGE NUMBER
15	17	177	35
18	57	202	27
29	109	208	22
35	153	216	32
43	54	223	72
46	18	226	33
94	23	230	217
95	106	234	43
120	48	239	50
124	19	240	82
149	60	244	50
150	194	246	152
154	110	250	75
162	139	253	183
164	21	256	178

Bibliography and Index of Primary Authors

With complete citations, abstract numbers, and page references.

ABSTRACT		PAGE
1	American Pharmaceutical Association. *Pharmacy and the Poor.* Washington, D.C., The Association, 1971.	40, 109
2	American Pharmaceutical Association. *White Paper on the Pharmacist's Role in Product Selection.* Washington, D.C., The Association, 1971.	139
3	Anonymous. Administrative profiles. Cost of pharmacy services. *Hospitals 43* (*16*):28, March 16, 1969.	92
4	Anonymous. California's volume purchase plan. *Pharmacy West 88* (*2*):51–66, February 1976.	145
5	Anonymous. The cost of drugs. *New Zealand Medical Journal 69* (*440*):33–34, January 1969.	80, 142
6	Anonymous. Drug substitutions. *Hospital Formulary Management 6* (*12*):29, December 1971.	140, 215
7	Anonymous. Evolution of the final Maximum Allowable Cost regulations. *Journal of the American Pharmaceutical Association NS15* (*9*):506–526, September 1975.	117
8	Anonymous. The formulary in your future. *Physician's Management 13* (*10*):33–34, 40, 42–44, 49, 53, October 1973.	212
9	Anonymous. How to pay less for prescription drugs. *Consumer Reports 40* (*1*):48–53, January 1975.	123
10	Anonymous. In 1968 . . . insurance paid an estimated $125 million for medications. *American Professional Pharmacist 35* (*3*):40–41, March 1969.	47
11	Anonymous. Limits on drug reimbursements to save millions. *Record 1* (*3*):13–17, June 1977.	113
12	Anonymous. Many oppose substitution, survey shows. *Drug Topics 119* (*12*):6, June 16, 1975.	124
13	Anonymous. Medicare-Medicaid: An appraisal after ten years. Special section of seven papers. *Public Health Reports 91* (4):299–342, July–August 1976.	5

14	Anonymous. Pharmaceutical industry. Price regulation scheme erroneously based, says Office of Health Economics report. *Pharmaceutical Journal 215* (*5834*):210, September 6, 1975.	64
15	Anonymous. *Revolution in Health Care.* Proceedings of a Symposium Held in Sacramento, California, September 8, 1975. Nutley, New Jersey, Hoffmann-LaRoche, 1976.	17
16	Anonymous. Source options in Health Maintenance Organization pharmacy service. *Hospitals 47* (*24*):75–77, December 16, 1973.	34
17	Apple, William S. Problems facing pharmacists under Medicare and Medicaid. *Journal of the American Pharmaceutical Association NS10* (*9*):494–500, September 1970.	44, 170
18	Bachynsky, J.A. Report from Canada. *In* Wertheimer, Albert I., Editor. *Proceedings of the International Conference on Drug and Pharmaceutical Services Reimbursement.* Public Health Service. Health Resources Administration. National Center for Health Services Research. DHEW Publication No. (HRA) 77-3186. Springfield, Virginia, National Technical Information Service, June 1977. Pages 73–83.	57
19	Bachynsky, John A.; and Hammel, Robert W. Under tax supported programs. Cost of providing pharmaceuticals. *Journal of the American Pharmaceutical Association NS9* (*6*):269–272, June 1969.	47
20	Bauer, Raymond A.; and Field, Mark G. Ironic contrast: United States and Union of Soviet Socialist Republics drug industries. *Harvard Business Review 40* (*5*):89–97, September–October 1962.	83
21	Berki, S.E.; Richards, J.W.; and Weeks, H.A. The mysteries of prescription pricing in retail pharmacies. *Medical Care 15* (*3*):241–250, March 1977.	13, 149
22	Billups, Norman F.; and McGee, L. Randolph. The relative stability of drug prices and pharmacists' fees. *Journal of the American Pharmaceutical Association NS11* (*1*):22–25, January 1971.	41
23	Blake, Martin I. Role of the compendia in controlling factors affecting bioavailability of drug products. *Journal of the American Pharmaceutical Association NS11* (*11*):603–611, November 1971.	140
24	Bower, Richard M.; and Hepler, Charles D. A statistical approach to per diem pharmacy pricing. *American Journal of Hospital Pharmacy 31* (*12*):1179–1188, December 1974.	89
25	Brandon, Brenda M.; Knapp, David A.; Klein, Linda S.; and Gregory, John. Drug usage screening criteria. *American Journal of Hospital Pharmacy 34* (*2*):146–151, February 1977.	173
26	Brewster, Agnes W.; Allen, Scott I.; and Holen, Arlene. Patterns of drug use by type in a prepaid medical plan. *Public Health Reports 79* (*5*):403–409, May 1964.	54
27	Brewster, Agnes W.; Allen, Scott I.; and Kramer, Lucy M. Experience with a prepaid drug benefit. *Journal of Health and Human Behavior 4* (*1*):14–22, Spring 1963.	55
28	Brewster, Agnes W.; and Horton, Juanita P. The relationship of drug costs to medical care. *American Journal of Hospital Pharmacy 25* (*4*):176–179, April 1968.	51

29	Brindle, James; and Wolman, Milton H. The prepaid group practice point of view. *Journal of the American Pharmaceutical Association NS11* (2):68–70, February 1971.	109
30	Brodie, Donald C. *Drug Utilization and Drug Utilization Review and Control.* Public Health Service, Health Services and Mental Health Administration. DHEW Publication No. (HSM) 72-3002. Washington, D.C., United States Government Printing Office, April 1970.	199
31	Brodie, Donald C.; and Smith, William E. Constructing a conceptual model of drug utilization review. *Hospitals 50* (6):143–144, 146, 148, 150, March 1976.	179
32	Brodie, Donald C.; Smith, William E.; and Hlynka, John N. Model for drug usage review in a hospital. *American Journal of Hospital Pharmacy 34* (3):251–254, March 1977.	173
33	Brook, Robert H.; and Williams, Kathleen N. Effect of medical care review on the use of injections. A study of the New Mexico experimental medical care review organization. *Annals of Internal Medicine 85* (4):509–515, October 1976.	180
34	Brooke, Paul A. *Resistant Prices: A Study of Competitive Strains in the Antibiotic Markets.* New York, Council on Economic Priorities, 1975.	125
35	Brooks, Geoffrey E.; and Knapp, David A. Economics of institutional pharmacy services under national health insurance in Australia. *American Journal of Hospital Pharmacy 32* (10):1018–1022, October 1975.	64, 153
36	Burack, Richard. *The New Handbook of Prescription Drugs: Official Names, Prices, and Sources for Patient and Doctor.* New York, Ballantine Books, 1970.	45, 142
37	Bush, Patricia J.; and Wertheimer, Albert I. Pharmacy and the Health Maintenance Organization—the British experience. *Journal of the American Pharmaceutical Association NS15* (12):691–695, 704, December 1975.	65
38	California Department of Health Care Services. *Medi-Cal: California Medicaid: A Management and Utilization Study.* Sacramento, The Department, 1970.	199
39	Canadian Pharmaceutical Association. *Pharmacy in a New Age.* Commission on Pharmaceutical Services. Toronto, The Association, 1971.	78
40	Carlova, John. Will Maximum Allowable Cost cut prescription costs? Let's take a good look! *Drug Topics 120* (4):39–40, February 15, 1976.	203
41	Castle, W.B.; Astwood, E.B.; Finland, Maxwell; and Keefer, Chester S. White paper on the therapeutic equivalence of chemically equivalent drugs. *Journal of the American Medical Association 208* (7):1171–1172, May 19, 1969.	143
42	Chewning, John B. New professional liability problems? Legal implications of generic drug substitution. *Ohio State Medical Journal 71* (5):323–326, May 1975.	125
43	Clapp, Raymond F. *Study of Drug Purchase Problems and Policies. Welfare Research Report 2.* United States Department of Health, Education, and Welfare. Washington, D.C., United States Government Printing Office, March 1966.	54

44 Comptroller General of the United States. *Controls over Medicaid Drug Program in Ohio Need Improvement.* Washington, D.C., Comptroller General, 1970. 46, 171

45 Comptroller General of the United States. *Review of Pricing Methods Used by Various States in the Purchase of Prescribed Drugs under Federally Aided Public Assistance Programs.* Report to the United States Congress. Washington, D.C., Comptroller General, 1967. 171

46 Conley, Bernard E. *Social and Economic Aspects of Drug Utilization Research.* Hamilton, Illinois, Drug Intelligence Publications, 1976. 18

47 Cotton, Hugh A.; and Rucker, T. Donald. Prescription cost determination in Kansas. *Journal of the American Pharmaceutical Association NS12* (*8*):412–415, August 1972. 163

48 Dardis, Rachel; and Dowdell, D. Price variations for prescription drugs. *Journal of Retailing 52* (*3*):15–26, Fall 1976. 18

49 DeNuzzo, Rinaldo V. Annual prescription survey by the Albany College of Pharmacy. *Medical Marketing and Media 12* (*4*):32–43, 46, 48–49, April 1977. 13

50 Dick, M. Lawrence; Winship, Henry W., III; and Wood, George C. A cost effectiveness comparison of a pharmacist using three methods for identifying possible drug related problems. *Drug Intelligence and Clinical Pharmacy 9* (*5*):257–262, May 1975. 86

51 Dickens, Paul F., III. *The Maximum Allowable Cost Regulations and Pharmaceutical Research and Development.* Research and Statistics Note. Note No. 2-1976. Office of Research and Statistics. Social Security Administration. DHEW Publication No. (SSA) 76-11701. Washington, D.C., United States Government Printing Office, March 4, 1976. 116

52 Dickens, Paul; and Hogan, Timothy D. *The Maximum Allowable Cost Program and Wholesale Drug Prices, a Preliminary Analysis.* Research and Statistics Note. Note No. 11. Washington, D.C., Social Security Administration, July 12, 1977. 114

53 Dickson, W. Michael; and Rodowskas, Christopher A., Jr. Research report. Allocation of pharmacist time for third-party prescription plans. *Inquiry 12* (*3*):263–267, September 1975. 153

54 Donabedian, Avedis. *Benefits in Medical Care Programs.* Cambridge, Massachusetts, Harvard University Press, 1976. 6

55 Donabedian, Avedis. Issues in national health insurance. *American Journal of Public Health 66* (*4*):345–350, April 1976. 6

56 Donabedian, Avedis; and Attwood, Julia C. An evaluation of administrative controls in medical care programs. *New England Journal of Medicine 269* (*7*):347–354, August 15, 1963. 10

57 Drug Quality and Therapeutics Committee. *PARCOST Comparative Drug Index.* Seventh Edition. Ottawa, Canada, Ministry of Health, 1974. 72, 128

58 Ellis, Robert F.; and Sice, Jean. Availability and cost of urinary antibacterials in a metropolitan area. *Journal of Chronic Diseases 26* (*10*):617–622, 1973. 34

59 Executive Office of the President. The problem of rising health care 7

costs. Council on Wage and Price Stability staff report. *Medical Marketing and Media 11* (*11*):42–47, 50, 52, 54–59, November 1976.

60 Feldmann, Edward G. Future of drug compendia. *Journal of the American Pharmaceutical Association NS15* (4):198–201, April 1975. 206

61 Finch, Dennis K. Opportunities for a prepaid pharmacy foundation. *Journal of the American Pharmaceutical Association NS12* (4):173–175, April 1972. 164

62 Fink, Joseph L., III. A community formulary for Delaware? *Delaware Medical Journal 62* (2):41–43, February 1970. 218

63 Fink, Joseph L., III. Some legal aspects of the hospital formulary system. *American Journal of Hospital Pharmacy 31* (*1*):86–90, January 1974. 209

64 Fletcher, Linda P. Prepaid drug plans sponsored by pharmacists. *Journal of Risk and Insurance 34* (*1*):81–94, March 1967. 53

65 Fletcher, Linda P.; Gagnon, Jean P.; and Rodowskas, Christopher A., Jr. Communications. *Journal of Risk and Insurance 41* (4):739–747, December 1974. 157

66 Follmann, J.F., Jr. Health insurance for the cost of drugs. *American Journal of Public Health 51* (5):659–664, May 1961. 56

67 Food and Drug Administration. *Holders of Approved New Drug Applications for Drugs Presenting Actual or Potential Bioequivalence Problems.* HEW Publication No. (FDA) 76-3009. Rockville, Maryland, Food and Drug Administration, June 1976. 120

68 Forman, Howard I. Drug patents, compulsory licenses, prices and innovation. *In* Cooper, Joseph D., Editor. *Economics of Drug Innovation.* Proceedings of the First Seminar on Economics of Pharmaceutical Innovation, April 1969. Washington, D.C., American University, 1970. Pages 177–198. 78, 146

69 Francke, Donald E. The formulary system: product of the teaching hospital. *Hospitals 41* (*22*):110, 112, 114, 116, November 16, 1967. 220

70 Friend, Dale G.; Goolkasian, A. Richardson; Hassan, William E., Jr.; and Vona, Joseph P. Generic terminology and the cost of drugs. *Journal of the American Medical Association 209* (*1*):80–84, July 7, 1969. 143

71 Fuchs, Victor R. Drugs. *In* Fuchs, Victor R. *Who Shall Live?* New York, Basic Books, 1974. Pages 120–124. 28

72 Fuchs, Victor R. From Bismarck to Woodcock: the "irrational" pursuit of national health insurance. *The Journal of Law and Economics 19* (2):347–359, August 1976. 8

73 Fulda, Thomas R. Drug cost control: The road to the maximum allowable cost regulations. *In* Friedman, Kenneth; and Rakoff, Stuart. *Toward a National Health Policy. Public Policy in the Control of Health Care Costs.* Lexington, Massachusetts, Lexington Books, 1977. Pages 55–67. 14, 114

74 Furstenberg, Frank F.; and Cline, Raleigh. The effect of a drug formulary on costs and quality of medical care in a public medical program. *In Tenth Annual Group Health Institute of Group Health Associations of America Proceedings.* Columbus, Ohio, The Institute, May 1960. Pages 167–179. 221

75	Gagnon, Jean P.; Nelson, Arthur A.; and Rodowskas, Christopher A., Jr. A comparison of maintenance and nonmaintenance outpatient prescription directions, durations of coverage and costs per day. *Medical Care 13* (*1*):47–58, January 1975.	23
76	Gagnon, Jean Paul; and Rodowskas, Christopher A., Jr. Reimbursement methods for pharmaceutical service. *Journal of the American Pharmaceutical Association NS14* (*12*):675–678, December 1974.	158
77	Gagnon, Jean P.; and Rodowskas, Christopher A., Jr. A study of the relationships of drug dosage form, therapeutic class and pharmaceutical services with the gross margins on prescription drugs. *Medical Care 12* (*1*):49–61, January 1974.	159
78	Gagnon, Jean P.; and Rodowskas, Christopher A., Jr. Two controversial problems in third-party outpatient prescription plans. *Journal of Risk and Insurance 39* (4):603–611, December 1972.	37, 165
79	Gardner, Vince. Maximum Allowable Cost-Estimated Acquisition Cost. The view from Washington. *California Pharmacist 24* (*1*):36–39, July 1976.	116
80	Garner, Dewey D., Editor. *Bibliography of Theses and Dissertations Relevant to Pharmacy Administration. 1970–1974.* Bethesda, Maryland, American Association of Colleges of Pharmacy, 1976.	19
81	Gibson, Tyrone. Generic equivalency and Food and Drug Administration approved usage. What are the true effects of drugs? *Hospital Formulary Management 9* (*11*):39, 42, 44, 46, 48–49, 54, 56, 58, November 1974.	128
82	Goldberg, Theodore; Aldridge, Gerald W.; DeVito, Carolee A.; Vidis, Jerry; Moore, Willis E.; and Dickson, W. Michael. Impact of drug substitution legislation: A report of the first year's experience. *Journal of the American Pharmaceutical Association NS17* (4):216–226, April 1977.	119
83	Goldberg, Theodore; and Loren, Eugene L. The United Auto Workers' negotiated prepaid prescription drug program. *Journal of the American Pharmaceutical Association NS12* (*8*):422–425, August 1972.	38, 101
84	Goldberg, Theodore; Moore, Willis E.; Koontz, Theodore; Facione, Frank; Aldridge, Gerald; Vidis, Jerry; Vadasy, Patricia; and Jones, Gail. Evaluation of impact of drug substitution legislation. *Journal of the American Pharmaceutical Association NS16* (2):64–70, 90, February 1976.	120
85	Gosselin, Raymond. Statement. *In* United States House of Representatives. *Hearings before the Subcommittee on Environmental Problems Affecting Small Business of the Select Committee on Small Business. Third-Party Prepaid Prescription Programs.* Ninety-second Congress. First Session. Washington, D.C., United States Government Printing Office, 1971. Pages 154–162.	166
86	Gosselin, R.A. and Company. *Pharmacy Charges for Prescription Drugs under Third-Party Programs. Variability Analysis. Final Report.* Dedham, Massachusetts, R.A. Gosselin and Company, 1971.	166
87	Greenlick, Merwyn R.; and Darsky, Benjamin J. A comparison of general drug utilization in a metropolitan community with utilization under a drug prepayment plan. *American Journal of Public Health 58* (*11*):2121–2136, November 1968.	81

88	Greenlick, Merwyn R.; and Saward, Ernest W. Impact of a reduced-charge drug benefit in a prepaid group practice plan. *Public Health Reports 81* (*10*):938–940, October 1966.	111
89	Gregory, John M.; and Knapp, Deanne E. State-of-the-art of drug usage review. *American Journal of Hospital Pharmacy 33* (*9*):925–928, September 1976.	180
90	Gulick, William. *Consumers' Guide to Prescription Prices.* Syracuse, Consumer Age Press, 1973.	135
91	Gumbhir, Ashok K.; and Rodowskas, Christopher A., Jr. Consumer price differentials between generic and brand name prescriptions. *American Journal of Public Health 64* (*10*):977–982, October 1974.	129
92	Hall, Nathan A. Pharmaceutical aspects of the Australian national health scheme. *Journal of the American Pharmaceutical Association NS9* (*4*):184–186, April 1969.	81, 219
93	Hammel, Robert W. Insights into public assistance medical care expenditures. *Journal of the American Medical Association 219* (*13*):1740–1744, March 27, 1972.	214
94	Harris, Seymour E. Drugs. *In* Harris, Seymour E. *The Economics of Health Care. Finance and Delivery.* Berkeley, California, McCutchan Publishing Corporation, 1975. Pages 255–263.	23
95	Health Services Administration. *Inclusion of Pharmaceutical Services in Health Maintenance and Related Organizations: A Review of Supplemental Benefits.* DHEW Publication No. (HSA) 74-13017. Washington, D.C., United States Government Printing Office, 1974.	106
96	Helfand, William H. The United States and international drug regulatory approaches. *Journal of the American Pharmaceutical Association NS15* (*12*):702–704, December 1975.	66
97	Helmer, Irmela. Report from West Germany. *In* Wertheimer, Albert I., Editor. *Proceedings of the International Conference on Drug and Pharmaceutical Services Reimbursement.* Public Health Service. Health Resources Administration. National Center for Health Services Research. DHEW Publication No. (HRA) 77-3186. Springfield, Virginia, National Technical Information Service, June 1977. Pages 29–36.	58
98	Hemminki, Elina. Review of literature on the factors affecting drug prescribing. *Social Science and Medicine 9* (*2*):111–116, February 1975.	24
99	Hennessy, William B. A fee-per-patient-per-day basis for delivering pharmaceutical services to an institution. *Journal of the American Pharmaceutical Association NS9* (*11*):561–562, November 1969.	92
100	Hirschman, Joseph L.; and Laventurier, Marc. Professional Standards Review Organizations—participation pathways for pharmacists. *Drug Intelligence and Clinical Pharmacy 9* (*10*):553–556, October 1975.	184
101	Hopkins, Carl E.; Roemer, Milton I.; Procter, Donald M.; Gartside, Foline; Lubitz, James; Gardner, Gerald A.; and Moser, Marc. Cost-sharing and prior authorization effects on Medicaid services in California: Part 1. The beneficiaries' reactions. *Medical Care 13* (*7*):582–594, July 1975.	98

102	Hopkins, Carl E.; Roemer, Milton I.; Procter, Donald M.; Gartside, Foline; Lubitz, James; Gardner, Gerald A.; and Moser, Marc. Cost-sharing and prior authorization effects on Medicaid services in California: Part II: The providers' reactions. *Medical Care 13* (*8*):643–647, August 1975.	98
103	Hornbrook, Mark C. A commentary on "The interdependence of prescription drugs and other health care costs": some implications for research. *Drugs in Health Care 2* (4):255–265, Fall 1975.	25
104	Horvitz, Richard A.; Morgan, John P.; and Fleckenstein, Lawrence. Savings from generic prescriptions. A study of 33 pharmacies in Rochester, New York. *Annals of Internal Medicine 82* (5):601–607, May 1975.	126
105	Hull, J. Heyward; Brown, H. Shelton; Yarborough, Frank F.; and Murray, William J. Drug utilization review of Medicaid patients: therapeutic implications and opportunities. *North Carolina Medical Journal 36* (*3*):162–163, March 1975.	185
106	Huskisson, E.C. Trade names or proper names?—A problem for the prescriber. *British Medical Journal* 4 (*5886*):225–228, October 27, 1973.	75, 135
107	IMS America. *National Prescription Audit. General Information Report.* Ambler, Pennsylvania, IMS America, Limited, 1974.	29
108	Iowa Department of Social Services. *Medicaid Drug Program Utilization Study.* Des Moines, Bureau of Medical Services, 1973.	190
109	Jacinto, Marcia S.; Kleinmann, Kurt; and Margolin, Joseph. Pharmacist-monitored, computerized drug usage review. *American Journal of Hospital Pharmacy 31* (5):508–512, May 1974.	189
110	Jødal, Bjørn. Report from Norway. *In* Wertheimer, Albert I., Editor. *Proceedings of the International Conference on Drug and Pharmaceutical Services Reimbursement.* Public Health Service. Health Resources Administration. National Center for Health Services Research. DHEW Publication No. (HRA) 77-3186. Springfield, Virginia, National Technical Information Service, June 1977. Pages 105–120.	58
111	Johnson, Richard E.; and Campbell, William H. Drug services and costs in Health Maintenance Organization prototypes. *American Journal of Hospital Pharmacy 30* (5):405–421, May 1973.	107
112	Johnson, Richard E.; Campbell, William H.; Azevedo, Daniel J.; and Drichas, Marilyn W. *Drug Utilization of a Four Year Cohort of HEW-Neighborhood Health Center Program Participants.* Portland, Oregon, Kaiser Foundation Hospitals, no date.	200
113	Jones, Donald J.; and Follman, J.F. *Health Insurance and Prescription Drugs.* Washington, D.C., Health Insurance Association of America, 1971.	41
114	Jones, I.F. Community pharmacy. Pharmacy and the National Health Service. Contractors' attitudes. *Pharmaceutical Journal 215* (*5831*):150–153, August 16, 1975.	67, 154
115	Jones, I.F. Community pharmacy. Pharmacy and the National Health Service. A proposed new charter for pharmacy. *Pharmaceutical Journal 215* (*5834*):211–214, September 6, 1975.	67, 155

116 Jones I.F.; and Booth, T.G. Pharmacy and the National Health Service. 1. Some basic issues. *Pharmaceutical Journal 215* (*5828*):72–74, July 26, 1975. 68, 156

117 Jones, I.F.; and Booth, T.G. Pharmacy and the National Health Service. 2. Macro-economic aspects and trends. *Pharmaceutical Journal 215* (*5829*):96–99, August 2, 1975. 69, 156

118 Kanig, Joseph L. Product selection: community formularies and legal aspects. *American Journal of Pharmacy 144* (5):133–138, September–October 1972. 138, 215

119 Karr, G. Monitoring drug utilization—modification of physician prescribing habits. *Canadian Journal of Hospital Pharmacy 30* (*1*):13–15, January–February 1977. 174

120 Kavaler, Florence; Bellin, Lowell E.; Green, Alex; Gorelik, Elihu A.; and Alexander, Raymond S. A publicly funded pharmacy program under Medicaid in New York City. *Medical Care 7* (5):361–371, September–October 1969. 48

121 Kelly, A.D. Drug costs under hospital insurance. *Canadian Medical Association Journal 97* (*8*):425–427, August 19, 1967. 83

122 Kemp, Bernard A.; and Moyer, Paul R. Equivalent therapy at lower cost. The oral penicillins. *Journal of the American Medical Association 228* (*8*):1009–1014, May 20, 1974. 129

123 Kennard, Lon; Laventurier, Marc; and Lang, Cheryl. Categorically needy and medically needy. Drug utilization among the aged and disabled. *Medical Marketing and Media 12* (2):31, 34, 36–38, February 1977. 15

124 Kennard, Lon H.; and Roden, Donald R. Dispensing patterns under third party programs. *Medical Marketing and Media 11* (5):44, 46–47, 50–51, May 1976 19

125 Kline, A. Burt. Will shortages of raw materials and rising prices hurt our chances for better health care? *Public Health Reports 90* (*1*):3–9, January–February 1975. 10

126 Knapp, David A., Editor. *Bibliography of Theses and Dissertations Relevant to Pharmacy Administration.* Silver Spring, Maryland, American Association of Colleges of Pharmacy, 1970. 46

127 Knapp, David A. The restrictive formulary and drug use review in a Medicare out-of-hospital prescription drug program. *NARD Journal 95* (*20*):14–16, October 15, 1973. 191, 212

128 Knapp, David A. Review article. Paying for outpatient prescription drugs and related services in third-party programs. *Medical Care Review 28* (*8*):826–859, August 1971. 167

129 Knapp, David A.; Brandon, Brenda M.; Knapp, Deanne E.; Klein, Linda S.; and Palumbo, Francis B. *Incorporating Diagnosis Into Drug Use Review Systems. Final Report.* Office of Economic Opportunity Project No. 31617. Baltimore, University of Maryland School of Pharmacy, 1975. 185

130 Knapp, David A.; Brandon, Brenda M.; Knapp, Deanne E.; Klein, Linda S.; Palumbo Francis B.; and Shah, Rohit. Incorporating diag- 174

nosis information into a manual drug use review system. *Journal of the American Pharmaceutical Association NS17* (2):103–106, February 1977.

131 Knapp, David A.; Brandon, Brenda M.; West, Sheila; and Leavitt, Dean E. Drug use review—a manual system. *Journal of the American Pharmaceutical Association NS13* (8):417–420, 433, August 1973. 192

132 Knapp, David A.; Knapp, Deanne E.; Brandon, Brenda M.; and West, Sheila. Development and application of criteria in drug use review programs. *American Journal of Hospital Pharmacy 31* (7):648–656, July 1974. 189

133 Knapp, David A.; Knapp, Deanne E.; and Brooks, Geoffrey E. Drug use in Australia and the United States as reflections of legislation and social attitudes. *Drug Intelligence and Clinical Pharmacy 11* (5):298–303, May 1977. 59

134 Knapp, David A.; and Palumbo, Francis B. Dollar costs of conducting drug use review. *Journal of the American Pharmaceutical Association NS17* (4):231–233, April 1977. 175

135 Knapp, Deanne E.; Crosby, Dianne L.; Morgan, Thomas F.; Lao, Chang S.; Kennedy, J. Stephen; and Dormer, Robert A. *Drug Use Analysis Methodologies.* Accession No. PB 260542/AS. Springfield, Virginia 22161, National Technical Information Service, 1976. 181

136 Knoben, James E. Drug utilization review. Current status and relationship to assuring quality medical care. *Drug Intelligence and Clinical Pharmacy 10* (4):222–228, April 1976. 182

137 Knoben, James E. The Professional Standards Review Organization program—its impact on the provision of drug-related services. *Journal of the American Pharmaceutical Association NS15* (11):614–615, 644, November 1975. 186

138 Kotzan, Jeffrey A.; Hunter, Robert H.; and Tindall, William N. A quantitative analysis of antisubstitution repeal. *Medical Marketing and Media 10* (5):18–20, May 1975. 69, 126

139 Lasagna, Louis. The pharmaceutical revolution: its impact on science and society. *Science 166* (3910):1227–1233, December 5, 1969. 49

140 Laventurier, Marc F. *Ambulatory Medicare Prescription Drug Study.* Social Security Administration Proposal. Burlingame, California, PAID Prescriptions, Incorporated, 1974. 100

141 Lee, Armistead M. Comparative approaches to cost constraints in pharmaceutical benefits programs. *In* Mitchell, Samuel A.; and Link, Emery A., Editors. *Impact of Public Policy on Drug Innovation and Pricing.* Proceedings of the Third Seminar on Pharmaceutical Public Policy Issues, December 1975. Washington, D.C., American University, 1976. Pages 115–170. 20, 63

142 Lee, Armistead M. Drug use data: a different perspective. *Journal of the American Medical Association 234* (12):1242–1244, December 22, 1975. 187

143 Lee, Armistead M. The interdependence of prescription drugs and other health care costs. *Drugs in Health Care 2* (2):75–85, Spring 1975. 25

144 Lee, Armistead M. A reply to Hornbrook. *Drugs in Health Care 2* (4):255–265, Fall 1975. 26

145 Lee, Philip R. The Task Force on Prescription Drugs: a review of problems, progress and possibilities. *Drug Information Journal 11* (*1*):7–10, March 1977. 15

146 Lee, William M. The peril of "non-peer peer review." *Illinois Medical Journal 144* (*6*):597–598, December 1973. 136

147 LeRoy, A.A.; Morse, M.L.; and McCormick, W.C. *Physicians' Responses to Peer Review and Drug Utilization Review Procedures of a Medicaid Drug Program.* Jacksonville, Florida, PAID Prescriptions, 1976. 181

148 Lönngren, Rune. Experiences of the new pharmacy system in Sweden. *Journal of the American Pharmaceutical Association NS15* (*7*):379–381, 405, July 1975. 70, 105

149 Lönngren, Rune. Report from Sweden. *In* Wertheimer, Albert I., Editor. *Proceedings of the International Conference on Drug and Pharmaceutical Services Reimbursement.* Public Health Service. Health Resources Administration. National Center for Health Service Research. DHEW Publication No. (HRA) 77-3186. Springfield, Virginia, National Technical Information Service, June 1977. Pages 61–71. 60

150 Maronde, Robert F. *Drug Utilization Review with On-Line Computer Capability. Selected Methodology and Findings from a Demonstration.* Social Security Administration. Office of Research and Statistics, Staff Paper No. 13. DHEW Publication No. (SSA) 73-11853. Washington, D.C., United States Government Printing Office, May 1972. 194

151 Maronde, Robert F.; Lee, Peter V.; McCarron, Margaret M.; and Seibert, Stanley. A study of prescribing patterns. *Medical Care 9* (*5*): 383–395, September–October 1971. 197

152 Massachusetts Department of Public Health. The Massachusetts drug formulary. *New England Journal of Medicine 285* (*4*):232–233, July 22, 1971. 216

153 May, Franklin E.; Stewart, Ronald B.; and Cluff, Leighton E. Drug utilization in the hospital: an evaluation of drug costs. *Drugs in Health Care 2* (*3*):139–152, Summer 1975. 87, 187

154 McCaffree, Kenneth M.; and Newman, Harold F. Prepayment of drug costs under a group practice prepayment plan. *American Journal of Public Health 58* (*7*):1212–1218, July 1968. 110

155 McCormick, William C.; and Hammel, Robert W. Pharmacists' and physicians' attitudes toward removal of the prohibition on brand substitution: A comparative study. *Medical Marketing and Media 7* (*10*):27–30, 35–37, October 1972. 138

156 McDonald, Clement J.; Murray, Raymond; Jeris, David; Bhargava, Bharat; Seeger, Jay; and Blevins, Lonnie. A computer-based record and clinical monitoring system for ambulatory care. *American Journal of Public Health 67* (*3*):240–245, March 1977. 176

157 Meyer, Marvin C.; Bates, Herbert, Jr.; and Swift, Robert G. Providing quality drugs economically. The role of state formularies. *Journal of the American Pharmaceutical Association NS14* (*12*):663–666, December 1974. 130, 210

158 Mitchell, Bridger M.; and Schwartz, William B. Strategies for 8

financing national health insurance: who wins and who loses. *New England Journal of Medicine 295* (*16*):866–871, October 1976.

159 Morgan, John P. Watching the monitors: "PAID" Prescriptions, fiscal intermediaries and drug utilization review. *New England Journal of Medicine 296* (*5*):251–256, February 1977. 176

160 Muller, Charlotte. Drug benefits in health insurance. *International Journal of Health Services* 4 (*1*):157–170, Winter 1974. 29

161 Muller, Charlotte; and Krasner, Melvin. Pharmacy purchasing, formularies, and prices paid for drugs: a survey of hospitals in southern New York State. *American Journal of Hospital Pharmacy 30* (*9*):781–789, September 1973. 90, 213

162 Muller, Charlotte; Stolley, Paul D.; and Becker, Marshall H. Controlling drug costs. *American Journal of Public Health 62* (*6*):755–756, June 1972. 38, 139

163 National Center for Health Statistics. *Health. United States 1975.* Health Resources Administration. DHEW Publication No. (HRA) 76-1232. Washington, D.C., United States Government Printing Office, 1976. 9

164 National Pharmaceutical Council. *Pharmaceutical Benefits under State Medical Assistance Programs.* Washington, D.C., The Council, 1976. 21

165 Nelson, Arthur A.; and Gagnon, Jean P. Physician acceptance of three proposed programs designed to reduce prescription prices. *Drugs in Health Care 1* (*1*):27–37, Summer 1974. 131, 211

166 Nithman, Charles J.; Parkhurst, Yale E.; and Sommers, E. Blanche. Physicians' prescribing habits. Effects of Medicare. *Journal of the American Medical Association 217* (*5*):585–587, August 2, 1971. 91

167 Nold, Edward G.; and Pathak, Dev S. Third-party reimbursement for clinical pharmacy services: philosophy and practice. *American Journal of Hospital Pharmacy 34* (*8*):823–826, August 1977. 150

168 Norwood, G. Joseph; Lipson, David P.; and Freeman, Robert A. Policy implications of Maximum Allowable Cost: Average Wholesale Price-Actual Acquisition Cost differentials among pharmacies. *Journal of the American Pharmaceutical Association NS17* (*8*):496–499, August 1977. 115

169 Office of Technology Assessment. *Drug Bioequivalence.* Washington, D.C., United States Government Printing Office, 1974. 132

170 Opit, L.J.; and Farmer, R.D.T. National health service. Cost of dispensing in the pharmaceutical services. *The Lancet 1* (*7849*):160, 162, February 2, 1974. 73, 160

171 PAID Prescriptions. *1970–71 Report on Administration of the Medi-Cal Drug Program for the San Joaquin Foundation for Medical Care on a Prepayment Basis.* San Mateo, California, PAID Prescriptions, no date. 200

172 Palumbo, Francis B.; Knapp, David A.; Brandon, Brenda M.; Knapp, Deanne E.; Solomon, David K.; Klein, Linda S.; and Shah, Rohit K. Detecting prescribing problems through drug usage review: a case study. *American Journal of Hospital Pharmacy 34* (*2*):152–154, February 1977. 177

173	Pearce, H.G. The economic impact of third party payment for drugs. *Medical Marketing and Media 4* (*11*):25–26, 28–29, November 1969.	49
174	Pharmaceutical Manufacturers Association. *Brands, Generics, Prices and Quality: The Prescribing Debate after a Decade.* Washington, D.C., The Association, 1971.	141
175	Pharmaceutical Manufacturers Association. *Multiple Brands of Prescription Drugs: Effects and Implications for Pharmacy Inventories.* Washington, D.C., The Association, July 1973.	136
176	Pharmaceutical Manufacturers Association. *National Health Program Survey of Eight European Countries.* Washington, D.C., The Association, 1970.	79
177	Pharmaceutical Manufacturers Association. *Pharmaceutical Payment Programs—An Overview: The Financing of Prescription Medicines through Third-Party Programs.* Washington, D.C., The Association, 1973.	35
178	Pharmaceutical Manufacturers Association. *Prescription Drug Industry. Factbook '76.* Washington, D.C., The Association, 1976.	21
179	Phelps, Charles E.; and Newhouse, Joseph P. Effect of coinsurance: a multivariate analysis. *Social Security Bulletin 35* (*6*):20–28, 44, June 1972.	102
180	Pierpaoli, Paul G.; Coarse, James F.; and Tilton, Richard C. Antibiotic use control—an institutional model. *Drug Intelligence and Clinical Pharmacy 10* (*5*):258–267, May 1976.	182
181	Provost, George P. The capitation system for pharmaceutical services. *American Journal of Hospital Pharmacy 30* (*6*):493, June 1973.	162
182	Reilly, Mary Jo. Drug utilization review by pharmacy and therapeutics committees. *American Journal of Hospital Pharmacy 30* (*4*):349–350, April 1973.	192
183	Riley, David A.; Braucher, Charles L.; and Kotzan, Jeffrey A. An analysis of the adequacy of Medicaid prescriptions. *Journal of the American Pharmaceutical Association NS13* (*10*):571–573, October 1973.	213
184	Robles, Ramon R.; and Winship, Henry W., III. Pharmacy involvement in the neighborhood health center environment. *American Journal of Hospital Pharmacy 29* (*1*):68–71, January 1972.	39, 108
185	Roemer, Milton I.; Hopkins, Carl E.; Carr, Lockwood; and Gartside, Foline. Copayments for ambulatory care: pennywise and pound foolish. *Medical Care 13* (*6*):457–466, June 1975.	99
186	Rolands, Thomas F.; and Williams, Robert B. How drugs attain formulary listing. *Hospitals 49* (*2*):87–89, January 16, 1975.	87, 206
187	Rosenberg, Stephen N.; Berenson, Louise B.; Kavaler, Florence; and Gorelik, Elihu A. Prescribing patterns in the New York City Medicaid program. *Medical Care 12* (*2*):138–151, February 1974.	30, 132
188	Rosenberg, Stephen N.; Gunston, Christine; Berenson, Louise; and Klein, Arlette. An eclectic approach to quality control in fee-for-service health care: the New York City Medicaid experience. *American Journal of Public Health 66* (*1*):21–30, January 1976.	183
189	Rosner, Martin, M. The financial effects of formularies in hospitals. *American Journal of Hospital Pharmacy 23* (*12*):673–675, December 1966.	93, 220

190 Rucker, T. Donald. Basic methods for optimizing the rational prescribing of psychoactive drugs. *Journal of Drug Issues 1* (*3*): 326–332, Fall 1971. 42, 198

191 Rucker, T. Donald. Drug insurance, formularies, and pharmacy. *Medical Marketing and Media 6* (*10*):11–12, 14, 16–18, October 1971. 216

192 Rucker, T. Donald. Drug use. Data, sources, and limitations. *Journal of the American Medical Association 230* (*6*):888–890, November 11, 1974. 30, 190

193 Rucker, T. Donald. Economic aspects of drug over use. *Medical Annals of the District of Columbia 42* (*12*):609–614, December 1973. 36

194 Rucker, T. Donald. Economic problems in drug distribution. *Inquiry 9* (*3*):43–50, September 1972. 40

195 Rucker, T. Donald. National health insurance and prescription benefits. *Drug Intelligence and Clinical Pharmacy 10* (*9*):529–533, 1976. 21

196 Rucker, T. Donald. Possible impact of government drug program on community pharmacies. *Journal of the American Pharmaceutical Association NS 11* (*6*):334–337, June 1971. 43

197 Rucker, T. Donald. Professional Standards Review Organizations and pharmacy. *Journal of the American Pharmaceutical Association NS 13* (*10*):568–570, 591, October 1973. 193

198 Rucker, T. Donald. Public policy considerations in the pricing of prescription drugs in the United States. *International Journal of Health Services 4* (*1*):171–179, Winter 1974. 31, 160

199 Rucker, T. Donald. Review of Pharmaceutical Manufacturers Association, "Pharmaceutical Payment Programs—an Overview." *Drugs in Health Care 1* (*1*):52–54, Summer 1974. 32

200 Rucker, T. Donald. Review of Victor I. Fuchs, "Who Shall Live?" *Drugs in Health Care 2* (4):266–268, Fall 1975. 27

201 Rucker, T. Donald. The role of computers in drug utilization review. *American Journal of Hospital Pharmacy 29* (*2*):128–134, February 1972. 196

202 Rucker, T. Donald. Role of the pharmaceutical industry in a dynamic health care system. *Drugs in Health Care 2* (*2*):86–95, Spring 1975. 27

203 Rucker, T. Donald; and Visconti, James A. Hospital formularies: organizational aspects and supplementary components. *American Journal of Hospital Pharmacy 33* (*9*):912–917, September 1976. 85, 204

204 Ruderman, A. Peter. The drug business in the context of Canadian health care programs. *International Journal of Health Services 4* (4):641–650, 1974. 74, 133

205 Schicke, R.K. The pharmaceutical market and prescription drugs in the Federal Republic of Germany: cross-national comparisons. *International Journal of Health Services 3* (*2*):223–236, Spring 1973. 76

206 Schnell, B.R. Pharmaceutical services under the British National Health Service. *Drugs in Health Care 2* (*1*):70–71, Winter 1975. 71, 99

207 Schroeder, Steven A.; Kenders, Kathryn; Cooper, James K.; and Piemme, Thomas E. Use of laboratory tests and pharmaceuticals. Variation among physicians and effect of cost audit on subsequent 194

use. *Journal of the American Medical Association 225* (*8*):969–973, August 20, 1973.

208 Schwartzman, David. *Innovation in the Pharmaceutical Industry.* Baltimore, Johns Hopkins University Press, 1976. 22, 121

209 Scitovsky, Anne A.; and McCall, Nelda. Coinsurance and the demand for physician services: four years later. *Social Security Bulletin 40* (*5*):19–27, May 1977. 97

210 Scitovsky, Anne A.; and Snyder, Nelda M. Effect of coinsurance on physician services. *Social Security Bulletin 35* (*6*):3–19, June 1972. 102

211 Sharpe, Thomas R.; and Smith, Mickey C. The substitution controversy: attitudes of pharmacists toward repeal of antisubstitution laws. *Drugs in Health Care 3* (*1*):19–34, Winter 1976. 122

212 Shields, Arthur. Report from Australia. *In* Wertheimer, Albert I., Editor. *Proceedings of the International Conference on Drug and Pharmaceutical Services Reimbursement.* Public Health Service. Health Resources Administration. National Center for Health Services Research. DHEW Publication No. (HRA) 77-3186. Springfield, Virginia, National Technical Information Service, June 1977. Pages 37–59. 60

213 Siecker, Bruce R. Comprehensive pharmacy cost-finding. The path to pharmacist satisfaction. *California Pharmacist 24* (*1*):18–19, July 1976. 150

214 Siecker, Bruce R. *A Multi-Site Implementation and Evaluation of the Uniform Cost Accounting System for Pharmacy.* Washington, D.C., American Pharmaceutical Association Foundation, 1976. 151

215 Siecker, Bruce R. The uniform cost accounting approach for pharmacy pricing decisions. *Journal of the American Pharmaceutical Association NS17* (4):208–212, April 1977. 150

216 Silverman, Milton; and Lee, Philip R. *Pills, Profits, and Politics.* Berkeley, University of California Press, 1974. 32

217 Silverman, Milton; and Lydecker, Mia. *Drug Coverage under National Health Insurance: The Policy Options.* National Center for Health Services Research. Research Report Series. DHEW Publication No. (HRA) 77-3189. Springfield, Virginia, National Technical Information Service, 1977. 16

218 Simanis, Joseph G. *National Health Systems in Eight Countries.* United States Department of Health, Education, and Welfare. Social Security Administration. Office of Research and Statistics. DHEW Publication No. (SSA) 75-11924. Washington, D.C., United States Government Printing Office, January 1975. 71

219 Simmons, Henry E. Professional Standards Review Organizations: an opportunity for pharmacy. *Drugs in Health Care 2* (*1*):3–7, Winter 1975. 188

220 Simon, Wayne A.; Thompson, Louis; Campbell, Stuart; and Lantos, Robert L. Drug usage review and inventory analysis in promoting rational parenteral cephalosporin therapy. *American Journal of Hospital Pharmacy 32* (*11*):1116–1121, November 1975. 88, 207

221 Slywka, Gerald W.A.; Ryan, Michael R.; Melikian, Armen P.; Meyer, Marvin C.; Bates, Herbert E.; and Whyatt, Phillip L. Relationship of 120

price to bioavailability for four multiple-source drug products. *Journal of the American Pharmaceutical Association NS17* (*1*):30–32, January 1977.

222 Smith, Mickey C. *Drugs and Pharmacy Services under the British National Health Service. Final Report.* Department of Health Care Administration. Social Security Administration Grant No. 56096. University, Mississippi, University of Mississippi, 1973. 77

223 Smith, Mickey C. Pharmacy in the United Kingdom. *Journal of the American Pharmaceutical Association NS15* (*12*):687–690, December 1975. 72

224 Smith, Mickey, C. Prescribing patterns, physician reactions, and economic effects of closed and open formularies. *In* Anonymous. *Revolution in Health Care.* Proceedings of a Symposium Held in Columbia, South Carolina, September 30, 1974. Nutley, New Jersey, Hoffmann-LaRoche, 1975. Pages 40–45. 208

225 Smith, Mickey C. Psychotropic and analgesic drug prescriptions for patients seeing multiple physicians in a Medicaid program. *Medical Marketing and Media 12* (*1*):26, 28, 30–31, 34, January 1977. 203

226 Smith, Mickey C.; and Garner, Dewey D. Effects of a Medicaid program on prescription drug availability and acquisition. *Medical Care 12* (*7*):571–581, July 1974. 33

227 Smith, Mickey C.; Jones, Ian; and Booth, T. Geoffrey. Professional and economic bases for pharmaceutical services under the British National Health Service. *Drugs in Health Care 1* (*2*):59–73, Fall 1974. 74, 161

228 Smith, Mickey, C.; Jones, Ian; and Booth, T. Geoffrey. Research report. Paying the pharmacist under the British National Health Service. *Inquiry 10* (*3*):57–64, September 1973. 77, 162

229 Smith, Mickey C.; and Rowland, Clayton R. *Effects of Closing a Medicaid Formulary on Prescribing Psychotherapeutic Drugs.* Department of Health Care Administration. University, Mississippi, University of Mississippi, no date (1975?). 208

230 Social and Rehabilitation Service. Medical Services Administration. *Medicaid. Payment of Reasonable Charges for Prescribed Drugs.* DHEW Publication No. SRS-MSA-196-1971. Washington, D.C., United States Government Printing Office, 1971. 168, 217

231 Social and Rehabilitation Service. Medical Services Administration. *Results of Medicaid Provider Review—Massachusetts.* Washington, D.C., Social and Rehabilitation Service, 1977. 17

232 Stewart, Raymond. The Michigan generic substitution law: a survey of opinion. *Medical Marketing and Media 10* (*5*):22–23, May 1975. 127

233 Stolar, Michael H. Conceptual framework for drug usage review, medical audit and other patient care review procedures. *American Journal of Hospital Pharmacy 34* (*2*):139–145, February 1977. 178

234 Stolley, Paul, D.; and Goddard, James, L. Prescription drug insurance for the elderly under Medicare. *American Journal of Public Health 61* (*3*):574–581, March 1971. 43

235 Strom, Brian L.; Stolley, Paul D.; and Brown, Torrey C. Drug anti- 133

substitution studies. I: Estimation of possible savings by repeal of anti-substitution laws. *Drugs in Health Care 1* (2):99–103, Fall 1974.

236 Strom, Brian L.; Stolley, Paul D.; and Brown, Torrey C. Drug anti-substitution studies. II: Evaluation of pharmacists' attitudes toward repeal of anti-substitution laws. *Drugs in Health Care 1* (2):104–107, Fall 1974. 134

237 Swift, Robert G.; and Ryan, Michael R. Potential economic effects of a brand standardization policy in a 1000-bed hospital. *American Journal of Hospital Pharmacy 32* (*12*):1242–1250, December 1975. 89, 209

238 Talley, Robert B.; and Laventurier, Marc F. *Drug Utilization and Peer Review in San Joaquin.* Presented before the American Association of Foundations for Medical Care, Sea Island, Georgia, August 28, 1972. 196

239 Task Force on Prescription Drugs. *Approaches to Drug Insurance Design. Background Papers.* Office of the Secretary. United States Department of Health, Education, and Welfare. Washington, D.C., United States Government Printing Office, 1969. 50

240 Task Force on Prescription Drugs. *Current American and Foreign Programs. Background Papers.* Office of the Secretary. United States Department of Health, Education, and Welfare. Washington, D.C., United States Government Printing Office, 1968. 82

241 Task Force on Prescription Drugs. *The Drug Makers and the Drug Distributors. Background Papers.* Office of the Secretary. United States Department of Health, Education, and Welfare. Washington, D.C., United States Government Printing Office, 1968. 52

242 Task Force on Prescription Drugs. *The Drug Prescribers. Background Papers.* Office of the Secretary. United States Department of Health, Education, and Welfare. Washington, D.C., United States Government Printing Office, 1968. 52, 219

243 Task Force on Prescription Drugs. *The Drug Users. Background Papers.* Office of the Secretary. United States Department of Health, Education, and Welfare. Washington, D.C., United States Government Printing Office, 1968. 52

244 Task Force on Prescription Drugs. *Final Report.* Office of the Secretary. United States Department of Health, Education, and Welfare. Washington, D.C., United States Government Printing Office, 1969. 50

245 Taubman, Albert H.; and Gosselin, Raymond A. The Massachusetts Drug Formulary Act. *Journal of the American Pharmaceutical Association NS16* (2):71–73, February 1976. 122, 205

246 Trapnell, Gordon R. On measuring the effect of state reimbursement policy on Medicaid spending for prescription drugs. *In* Mitchell, Samuel A.; and Link, Emery A., Editors. *Impact of Public Policy on Drug Innovation and Pricing.* Proceedings of the Third Seminar on Pharmaceutical Public Policy Issues, December 1975. Washington, D.C., American University, 1976. Pages 195–222. 152

247 United States Department of Health, Education, and Welfare, Public Health Service. *Forward Plan for Health—Fiscal Years 1978–82.* Washington, D.C., The Department, August 1976. 9

248 United States House of Representatives. *Hearings before the Subcom-* 169

mittee on Environmental Problems Affecting Small Business of the Select Committee on Small Business. Third Party Prepaid Prescription Programs. Ninety-second Congress. First Session. Washington, D.C., United States Government Printing Office, 1971.

249 United States Senate. Special Committee on Aging. Subcommittee on Long-Term Care. *Nursing Home Care in the United States: Failure in Public Policy. Supporting Paper No. 2: Drugs in Nursing Homes: Misuse, High Costs, and Kickbacks.* Ninety-fourth Congress. First Session. Washington, D.C., United States Government Printing Office, 1975. — 28, 157

250 Wardell, William M. Control of drug utilization in the context of a national health service: the New Zealand system. *Clinical Pharmacology and Therapeutics 16* (*3*):585–594, September 1974. — 75

251 Weeks, H. Ashley. Changes in prescription drug utilization after the introduction of a prepaid drug insurance program. *Journal of the American Pharmaceutical Association NS13* (*4*):205–209, April 1973. — 100

252 Weinberger, Caspar W. Maximum allowable cost program—a closeup look. *Journal of the American Pharmaceutical Association NS15* (*7*):376–377, July 1975. — 118

253 Weissman, Alan M.; Solomon, David K.; Baumgartner, R. Paul, Jr.; Brady, Jeffrey A.; Peterson, James H.; and Knight, Joseph L. Computer support of pharmaceutical services for ambulatory patients. *American Journal of Hospital Pharmacy 33* (*11*):1171–1175, November 1976. — 183

254 Wertheimer, Albert I., Editor. *Proceedings of the International Conference on Drug and Pharmaceutical Services Reimbursement.* Public Health Service. Health Resources Administration. National Center for Health Services Research. DHEW Publication No. (HRA) 77-3186. Springfield, Virginia, National Technical Information Service, June 1977. — 61

255 Wertheimer, Albert I.; and Knoben, James E. The mail-order prescription drug industry. *Health Services Reports 88* (*9*):852–856, November 1973. — 36, 107

256 West, Sheila K.; Brandon, Brenda M.; Stevens, Anne M.; Zauber, Ann; Chase, Gary; Stolley, Paul D.; and Rumrill, Richard E. Drug utilization review in a Health Maintenance Organization. 1. Introduction and examples of methodology. *Medical Care 15* (*6*):505–514, June 1977. — 178

257 Whittet, T.D. Report from the United Kingdom. *In* Wertheimer, Albert I., Editor. *Proceedings of the International Conference on Drug and Pharmaceutical Services Reimbursement.* Public Health Service. Health Resources Administration. National Center for Health Services Research. DHEW Publication No. (HRA) 77-3186. Springfield, Virginia, National Technical Information Service, June 1977. Pages 85–103. — 62

258 Wolfe, Harvey. How cost-effective are generics? *Hospitals 47* (*9*):100, 104, 106, 108, May 1, 1973. — 91, 137

259 Zax, Brian B.; and Knapp, Deanne E. *Drug Use Analysis Bibliography.* Accession No. PB 264222/AS. Springfield, Virginia 22161, National Technical Information Service, March 1977. — 179

Index of Secondary Authors

Cross-referenced to primary authors and abstract numbers.

Subject Index

Numbers refer to pages, not abstracts